Karl-Heinz Schriever, Markus Schröder
G3P – Good Privacy Protection Practice in Clinical Research

Also of Interest

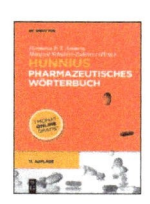

Hunnius Pharmazeutisches Wörterbuch
Hermann P. T. Ammon, Manfred Schubert-Zsilavecz (Hrsg.),
11. Aufl., 2014
ISBN: 978-3-11-030990-4

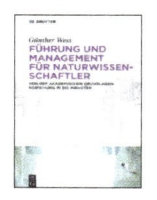

Führung und Management für Naturwissenschaftler
Von der akademischen Grundlagenforschung in die Industrie
Günther Wess, 2013
ISBN 978-3-11-031163-1, e-ISBN: 978-3-11-031168-6

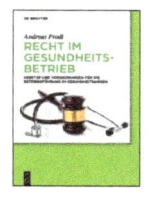

Recht im Gesundheitsbetrieb
Gesetze und Verordnungen für die Betriebsführung im
Gesundheitswesen
Andreas Frodl, 2013
ISBN: 978-3-11-033370-1, e-ISBN: 978-3-11-033558-3

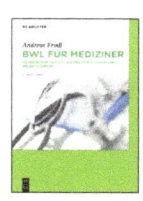

BWL für Mediziner
Betriebswirtschaftslehre für Studium und Selbststudium
Andreas Frodl, 2013
ISBN: 978-3-11-031345-1, e-ISBN: 978-3-11-031482-3

Karl-Heinz Schriever,
Markus Schröder

G3P – Good Privacy Protection Practice in Clinical Research

―

Principles of Pseudonymization and Anonymization

DE GRUYTER

Authors

Dr. Karl-Heinz Schriever
Eschenweg 3
88441 Mittelbiberach
E-mail: schriever-mittelbiberach@t-online.de

Markus Schröder
Tembit Software GmbH
Am Borsigturm 42
13507 Berlin
E-mail: schroeder@tembit.de

ISBN 978-3-11-055436-6
e-ISBN 978-3-11-028328-0
Set-ISBN 978-3-11-028329-7

Library of Congress Cataloging-in-Publication data
A CIP catalog record for this book has been applied for at the Library of Congress.

Bibliographic information published by the Deutsche Nationalbibliothek
The Deutsche Nationalbibliothek lists this publication in the Deutsche Nationalbibliografie; detailed bibliographic data are available on the Internet at http://dnb.dnb.de.

© 2017 Walter de Gruyter GmbH, Berlin/Boston
This volume is text- and page-identical with the hardback published in 2014.
Typesetting: fidus Publikations-Service GmbH, Nördlingen
Printing and binding: CPI books GmbH, Leck
Cover image: Purestock/Getty Images
♾ Printed on acid-free paper
Printed in Germany

www.degruyter.com

Preface

Protecting the privacy of personal data, safeguarding the individual freedom is one of the great challenges of today's democratic societies.

In our digitized world people often walk carelessly through the World Wide Web, revealing great parts of their privacy without being aware of potential unexpected and harmful effects and risks. Companies try to track information of web visitors in order to better judge the consumer behavior and thus to better adjust their market strategies.

Prospective employers used to ask applicants for a hand written curriculum vitae with the expectation that a subsequent analysis would reveal basic characteristics of potential candidates. Nowadays some employers ask for a genetic testing, and applicants often agree because they fear that a respective refusal could considerably decrease their chances of being hired.

The individual subject is often unable to cope with such tasks and challenges. It is the primary duty of the legislative authorities to implement a bundle of measures, a legal framework, guaranteeing that privacy will not be breached. Nevertheless, in the first instance it is up to you to take on responsibility for your personal data.

Establishing ethical and privacy protection aspects in scientific research, especially in medical research, has a long history. Medical data are usually more sensitive than other personal data and therefore require an even higher degree of protection. In recent research projects genetic evaluations have become more and more important and thereby trigger new and continuing activities in the context of data protection. Genetic data as a subset of medical data are the most sensitive category of personal data and require therefore the highest degree of data protection.

The book provides a systematic and itemized approach to data protection in clinical research including the handling of genetic material, genetic samples as well as derived genetic data and the subsequent secure storage of them. The set-up of different kinds of clinical trials having in addition a genetic part, the concept of a genetic informed consent as well as collection schemes of samples are described in detail.

Technical requirements and aspects of data protection including pseudonymization and anonymization procedures taking into account ethics committees requirements as well as the underlying legal framework are also presented.

Results of clinical trials submitted to regulatory authorities must have been derived by using validated environments. For readers who have never heard of validation we provide a brief introduction to the basic ideas and principles of validation. For those who are familiar with validation, and/or having already applied validation principles our explanations are primarily thought as a reminder.

An itemized description of the evaluation process of clinical and related genetic data is given, based on a sophisticated request management, including the establishment of an internal Genetic Review Board as counterpart to the external Ethics Committees.

To better understand the single steps of the data protection process we provide a brief but nevertheless itemized history of data protection in Europe and the U.S.

The guiding idea of data protection in the clinical environment is the principle of clinical Informed Consent. When conducting, however, clinical trials having also a supplementary genetic part, we must add a separate genetic Informed Consent, because participation in a clinical trial with genetic part as well as a possible withdrawal from either parts must be handled independently of each other. Descriptions of the mandatory sections of a genetic Informed Consent as well as proposals for their contents are presented in addition. A review of the related legal framework is an integral part of this chapter, too.

To support the individual data protection initiatives, a detailed listing of data protection and medical sites of interest has been prepared so that the reader can access these sites in the future to keep himself up to date.

Commissioned services like sample registration with and without relabeling, DNA extraction, biobanking, and statistical evaluations may have a high impact on the measures to be applied for anonymization and/or for preventing subjects from breaching anonymization. Sources of possible risks are identified, and respective measures to overcome those weaknesses are described and visualized by itemized workflow diagrams.

A practical guidance to clinical trials with genetic aspects is provided as a step by step approach in the following chapter. Detailed checklists are prepared, covering all aspects of a clinical trial with a supplementary genetic part, from the first idea up to the final evaluation of results, taking into account internal as well as external resources at each trial stage.

Some more material to extend the competent knowledge, acquired so far, is provided in the appendices 1 to 5 with respect to *Data Protection in the European Union*, *Data Types*, *Protection Masks*, *Informed Consent*, and *Security*.

Without any exception, all principles and methods presented are best practices, repeatedly applied in different clinical environments and by no means theoretical considerations.

The authors

Table of contents

About the Authors —— XI

1 Introduction —— 1

2 **Study Modes** —— 3
2.1 Screening Mode – Pharmacogenetic Information for Screening —— 3
2.2 Pre- Unspecified Mode – Pharmacogenetic as Part of a Study —— 3
2.3 Possible Approaches, Summary – Clinical Trial With Genetic Part —— 4
2.4 Biobanks – What do we Mean by That? —— 7

3 **Protection Masks and Procedures** —— 9
3.1 Identified Samples/Data —— 9
3.2 De-identified Samples/Data —— 10
3.3 Anonymized Samples/Data —— 10
3.4 Re-identification —— 11

4 **Coding Methods for De-identified Samples/Data** —— 13
4.1 Single-coded Samples/Data —— 13
4.2 Double-coded Samples/Data —— 14
4.3 Triple-coded Samples/Data —— 15

5 **Relationships Among the Protection Masks** —— 17

6 **Data Types** —— 19

7 **Anonymization** —— 23
7.1 Basic Terms and Ideas —— 23
7.2 Masking —— 24
7.3 Discarding the Key —— 30
7.4 Maintaining the Reliability of Stored Data —— 35
7.5 Security Measures —— 37

8 **Validation – a Brief Introduction** —— 43
8.1 Preliminaries —— 43
8.2 Basic Definitions & Terms —— 43
8.3 General Principles of Computer System Validation —— 45
8.4 Primary Validation – Specification Phase —— 47
8.5 Primary Validation – Preparing Operational Use —— 51
8.6 Primary Validation – Testing Phase —— 58

9 Request Management —— 67
9.1 Genetic Review Board (GRB) —— 67
9.2 Request Specification —— 68
9.3 Subrequest Specification —— 71
9.4 Involvement of External Service Providers —— 72

10 Legal Requirements & Regulations —— 75
10.1 Basic Ideas —— 75
10.2 Data Protection in the European Union (EU) —— 76
10.3 Transfer of Personal Data to Third Countries —— 92
10.4 Binding Corporate Rules —— 99
10.5 Data Protection in the United States (U.S.) – a Brief History —— 102

11 Informed Consent —— 109
11.1 Sections Mandatory for a Genetic Informed Consent —— 117

12 Selected Data Protection & Medical Sites —— 125
12.1 Germany —— 125
12.2 Europe —— 126
12.3 US —— 128
12.4 Global Initiatives —— 130

13 Impact of External Services on Data Protection —— 133
13.1 Introduction —— 133
13.2 Scenario 1 – Using GDI Throughout —— 135
13.3 Scenario 2 – Replacing GDI by nGDI Upon Sample Registration, Performed by regCRO —— 136
13.4 Scenario 3 – Replacing GDI by nGDI Upon Sample Registration, Performed by Sponsor —— 137
13.5 Scenario 4 – Sample Registration by CRO, Proprietary Labeling with CROSID —— 137
13.6 Scenario 5 – Barcoded Label bSID at Study Site —— 138
13.7 Overall Summary —— 139
13.8 External Statistical Evaluation —— 140
13.9 External Biobanking —— 140

14 Practical Approach to Clinical Trials with Supplementary Genetic Parts — 141
14.1 Introduction — 141
14.2 Overall Project Topology — 143
14.3 Checklist – Trial Set-up — 144
14.4 Checklist – System Topology — 146
14.5 Checklist – Sample Management — 146
14.6 Checklist – ICs, Ethics Committees Restrictions — 148
14.7 Checklist – Anonymization — 149
14.8 Checklist – Statistical Evaluation — 150

15 Appendix 1: Data Protection in the European Union — 153
15.1 Council of Europe (COE) — 153
15.2 EU Privacy Directive – Definitions — 153
15.3 Tasks of the Article 29 Data Protection Working Party — 154

16 Appendix 2: Data Types — 157
16.1 EU Privacy Directive (October 24, 1995) — 157
16.2 Council of Europe (COE) Definition of Data Types — 157
16.3 Federal Data Protection Act (GER) as of 1. Jan. 2003 — 160

17 Appendix 3: Protection Masks — 161
17.1 EMA definition of anonymous sample/data — 161
17.2 Germany — 161
17.3 Spain — 162
17.4 US — 163

18 Appendix 4: Informed Consent (IC) — 167
18.1 The Nuremberg Code — 167
18.2 EU Privacy Directive (October 24, 1995) — 168
18.3 COE – Rec No. R (97) 5, Explanatory Memorandum to Rec (97) 5 — 169
18.4 Oviedo Convention — 174
18.5 UNESCO Universal Declaration on Bioethics and Human Rights — 175
18.6 Key Issues in Informed Consent for Pharmacogenomics Research — 176
18.7 International Declaration On Human Genetic Data — 178
18.8 CIOMS – Ethical Guidelines for Biomedical Research — 179
18.9 Human Genetic Examination Act (Genetic Diagnosis Act – GenDG) — 181

19 Appendix 5: Security —— 185

19.1 EU Privacy Directive (October 24, 1995) —— 185
19.2 Federal Data Protection Act (Germany) —— 185
19.3 Council of Europe Recommendation No. R (97) 5 —— 186
19.4 US – Privacy Act of 1974 (Comments from William W. Lowrance, cf. (42)) —— 187
19.5 Safe Harbor Privacy Principles (2000) —— 188
19.6 UN – ICCPR International Covenant on Civil and Political Rights —— 188

20 Abbreviations —— 189

Anonymization —— 189
General —— 189

21 References —— 191

Index —— 197

About the Authors

Dr. Karl-Heinz Schriever
Dipl.-Math. Karl-Heinz Schriever, born October 27, 1948, looks back on more than forty years continuing experience in Medical Statistics and Medical Informatics. Starting his career at Karlsruhe University, his early interest was mainly in the development of sequential medical trials under ethical considerations. The practical implementation of statistical and computerized processes in industry has been widely performed during his employment as head of Biometry, Luitpold Werk, Munich, and Head of Informatics Medicine of Boehringer Ingelheim Pharma GmbH & Co. KG. Under his direction a broad spectrum of computerized systems necessary to successfully work in a medical environment within pharmaceutical industry has been specified, developed, and implemented, taking into account the advanced requirements of data protection in the medical field.

In recent years, Karl-Heinz Schriever focused mainly on the development and implementation of systems for biomedical research offering different approaches of a common statistical evaluation of clinical and related genetic data, and meeting all requirements of national and international data protection laws and regulations.

Since 2002 Karl-Heinz Schriever is lecturing on Mathematics and Statistics at the University of Applied Sciences at Biberach.

Dipl.-Inform. Markus Schröder
Dipl.-Inform. Markus Schröder, born March 29, 1960, is one of two founders of Tembit Software GmbH, Berlin, Germany (1992). Markus Schröder is head of the Healthcare Applications Department mainly focusing on the specification, development, and implementation of internet and telemedicine applications meeting highly sophisticated requirements with respect to security and data protection of medical and particularly genetic data.

Beginning with his early academic studies, Markus Schröder has been primarily concentrated on the realization of complete program suites in medical data processing, meeting the highest standards of data protection and data security of national and international laws and regulations.

Tembit realizes open source based, secure internet applications like generic electronic patient records, pseudonymization, anonymization and coding tools, as well as clinical study related genetic data handling applications.

Markus Schröder is an experienced specialist in managing large projects with international pharmaceutical companies, CROs, and university hospitals. The main objective of every Tembit healthcare application is the creation of reliable, completely validated systems, including 21 CFR Part 11 approval (electronic records and electronic signatures), having a high degree of sensitivity with respect to collected patient related data.

The high standard of Tembit's internet applications has been appreciated by granting the Open Source Best Practice Award in 2004, and multiple national and international data protection certificates thereafter.

Since 2010 Markus Schröder is Member of the Board of the National Association for eHealth Systems and Telemedicine (NEST), Germany.

1 Introduction

When evaluating clinical data and related samples from patients within a clinical trial, we are subjected to the Good Clinical Practice (GCP) principles, i.e. we are accustomed to provide a certain and appropriate degree of privacy with respect to the results of that trial (cf. (1)).

> **Guideline for good clinical practice E6 (R1)**
> **2.11** The confidentiality of records that could identify subjects should be protected, respecting the privacy and confidentiality rules in accordance with the applicable regulatory requirement(s).

Now that the genetic mapping technologies have gradually become so revealing, dealing with genetic data requires an even higher degree of privacy to be provided to all steps of the clinical trial process, especially to the results obtained. We are becoming more and more able to identify genetic factors that may indicate increased risks of diseases but are not uniquely the determinants of diseases. These new possibilities of predicting the development of diseases did simultaneously trigger ethical and legal initiatives toward solutions that will protect individuals against the use of genetic data against their interests, e.g. for the aptitude for employment, insurances for health and life as well as credit-worthiness (cf. (2), (3)).

These thoughts provide only a few arguments why genetic data are considered to be highly sensitive and thus require a different approach with respect to the data protection process as is usually implemented in the context of clinical data only. The special status of human genetic data has been already emphasized in Article 4 of the International Declaration on Human Genetic Data (cf. (4))

> **Article 4: Special status**
> (a) Human genetic data have a special status because:
> (i) they can be predictive of genetic predispositions concerning individuals;
> (ii) they may have a significant impact on the family, including offspring, extending over generations, and in some instances on the whole group to which the person concerned belongs;
> (iii) they may contain information the significance of which is not necessarily known at the time of the collection of the biological samples;
> (iv) they may have cultural significance for persons or groups.

There are numerous publications all focusing on the topics and terms arising in the context of genetic data processing, but there is no common terminology yet in that upcoming new field of clinical trial data processing; "the most universal quality is diversity", (Michel de Montaigne). Even the same terms are defined differently by various sources, and only few regulations are available that cover the area of handling genetic data within clinical trials. (cf. (5), (6), (7), (8))

Bear in mind that authorities in general publish only very few regulations. Most of the publications are conceived as guidances containing nonbinding recommendations. Nevertheless, those recommendations are widely understood as a broad hint how authorities expect procedures to be implemented.

New procedures must meet the recommendations of authorities to be considered as implicit regulations, as well as the needs of industry itself. An important additional factor that must not be underestimated and that must be considered before coming to a final decision is the public opinion.

It might be a wise decision if the procedures being implemented provide a certain degree of conformity with the public opinion with respect to the sensitive area of handling genetic data.

Possibly the decision to be taken is a balance between rational necessities on the one hand and political/public expectations on the other hand.

In any case, procedures to be implemented must allow adjustments to upcoming new regulations without major efforts.

When working in this context your interest should be focused on but not be limited to the following topics:
- Agreed Terminology in genetic data processing,
  i.e. unambiguously define the terms you use.
- Relevant Legal Requirements, laws, directives, regulations,
  i.e. be informed about legal requirements and/or boundaries that must be taken into account.
- Data Protection – protect the privacy of personal data,
  i.e. develop sensitivity and respective measures to guarantee a necessary and high level of data protection.
- Data Security – control the access to personal data,
  i.e. protect the physical security of personal data, adjust data security measures to the actual standards.
- Informed Consent for the participation in the clinical as well as in the genetic part of a clinical study – agreement which evaluations may be performed.

In addition, processes must be in place to handle:
- withdrawals from either part of a clinical study, clinical as well as genetic one at any time and if ever possible,
- and survey the workflow of samples collected for genetic analysis,
- possible restrictions to genetic analysis required most likely by Ethics Committees resp. IRBs,
- the coding or anonymization of data and samples,
- the secure storage of genetic data, original as well as derived data,
- requests for a common statistical analysis of coded (e.g. anonymized) clinical and related genetic data.

2 Study Modes

Prior to starting a clinical trial intended to have a genetic part, there must be a clear concept about which role genetics should play within the upcoming trial.

Four different approaches are currently imaginable:

2.1 Screening Mode – Pharmacogenetic Information for Screening

If genetic information is only used in order to select patients to be enrolled in a clinical study, we usually speak of **Screening Mode**, because patients are screened according to some genetic pattern, and the verification of a special pattern is mandatory for inclusion in the planned study.

The decision process when using screening mode is visualized in Fig. 2.1.

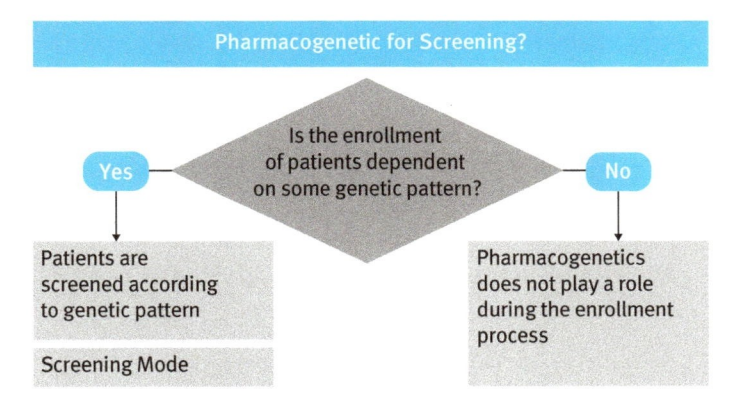

Fig. 2.1 Study Screening Opportunities

2.2 Pre-Unspecified Mode – Pharmacogenetic as Part of a Study

When planning to supplement the clinical part of a study by some kind of genetic analysis, two cases must be distinguished:
- We know for certain, prior to the start of the study, which kind of genetic analysis (genetic tests) should be performed.
  In this case, all genetic tests to be carried out must be prespecified in the Clinical Trial Protocol (CTP). We speak of **Prespecified Mode**.
- We do not know for certain, prior to the start of the study, which kind of genetic analysis should be performed.

In this situation we cannot specify genetic tests to be carried out in the CTP, i.e. genetic tests to be carried out later remain unspecified at that moment. Therefore, we speak of **Unspecified Mode**.

The decision process when to use which mode is visualized in Fig. 2.2.

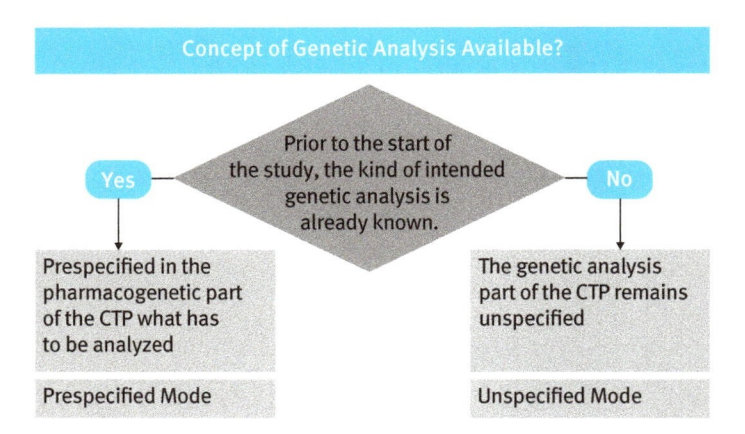

Fig. 2.2 Opportunities, if Genetic Analysis is Defined

Is it possible to apply both modes within one study?
Yes, it is.
- If you have a concrete idea with respect to genetic analysis, start with prespecified mode,
and
if you think there could be some more genetic analysis needed in the future, collect additional samples for later analysis (unspecified mode).

What does this mean in practice, how to proceed?
- Prespecified Mode – essentially „business as usual".
- Unspecified Mode – anonymization of data and samples is required prior to the start of a genetic analysis (cf. later).

2.3 Possible Approaches, Summary – Clinical Trial With Genetic Part

There are four possible approaches to supplement a clinical study with a genetic part (Fig. 2.3):
- If the genetic part is used as inclusion criteria, i.e. the verification of a specific genetic pattern is needed for the inclusion of a subject, you have to apply **Screening Mode (genotyping)**

- If you know in advance (prior to the start of the study), which genetic tests are to be evaluated later, you apply
  Prespecified Mode
- If you do not want or cannot specify in advance which genetic tests are to be evaluated later, then samples are collected, the DNA is extracted and stored for later analysis. You have to apply
  Unspecified Mode
- If you know in advance (prior to the start of the study), which genetic tests are to be evaluated later, and if you want to collect in addition samples for later analysis, then you have to apply
  Prespecified Mode on the first stage, and
  Unspecified Mode on the second stage

Screening Mode	A well defined genetic pattern is used as inclusion criterion.
Prespecified Mode	Genetic tests to be performed have been specified prior to the start of the respective clinical study.
Unspecified Mode	Genetic tests to be performed have not been specified prior to the start of the respective clinical study.
Pre- and Unspecified Mode	Combination of prespecified and unspecified mode.

Fig. 2.3 Alternative Study Modes

When applying prespecified mode, the following facts should be known:
- A trace back to the patient's identity is possible, but only the investigator knows the patient's identity.
- Data (clinical as well as genetic data) are de-identified by a code, e.g. PAT_NO (Patient Number).
- Essentially, samples will be destroyed after reporting of results.
- Genetic data analysis can be part of a submission.
- Source Data Verification (SDV) is possible due to the prespecified approach (de-identification of data).

Applying unspecified mode, the following facts should be known:
- A trace back to the patient's identity is not possible.
- Clinical data as well as genetic data are anonymized, the relationship of both data sources has been retained, but the relationship to the original PAT_NO has been broken.
- Samples are long-term stored in a biobank, preferably at least 10 years, if legally allowed.

- Genetic data analysis can be only supportive for a submission.
- SDV is not possible, due to anonymization.

Applying prespecified mode means that all genetic tests intended to be performed must be specified in the Clinical Trial Protocol and authorized by the competent Ethics Committees. Genetic tests not being prespecified must not be carried out, i.e. you are allowed to perform only those genetic tests that have been specified and authorized prior to the start of the study. Nothing more is allowed, even if you observe during genetic testing that some more genetic testing would be meaningful and worthwhile.

How to escape from this apparent impasse? Well, the most obvious solution would be to specify further genetic tests and to ask the competent Ethics Committees again for authorization. Most obvious but absolutely not feasible more often than not. Bear in mind that the layout of clinical trials generally covers a multitude of countries and centers within countries and thus a multitude of Ethics Committees concerned. An authorization of supplementary genetic tests in due time is hardly to achieve, if no resources for this additional project tasks have been budgeted in advance. The only way out of this situation is:
- to plan a more itemized, always well justified genetic testing. But bear in mind that an "omnibus authorization" is hardly achievable,

or
- to plan *Prespecified Mode* on the first stage and *Unspecified Mode* on the second stage from the outset of the respective project.

The second approach would enable you to perform additional genetic tests, however only with the anonymized samples. These supplementary genetic tests are not subject to authorization by competent Ethics Committees, but subject to authorization by your local Genetic Review Board (cf. chap. 9, Request Management).

Seeking for new scientific findings usually means research, and this conclusion in turn means that anonymization is the appropriate instrument, whenever possible. Compare e.g. the following section 40 of the BDSG, Germany.

> **Section 40 Processing and use of personal data by research institutions**
> (1) Personal data collected or recorded for purposes of scientific research may be processed or used only for purposes of scientific research.
> (2) Personal data shall be rendered anonymous as soon as the research purpose allows. Until then, the features enabling the attribution of information concerning personal or material circumstances to an identified or identifiable person shall be kept separately. They may be combined with the information only to the extent required by the research purpose.
> (3) Bodies conducting scientific research may publish personal data only if
> 1. the data subject has consented,
> 2. this is essential to present research findings concerning events of contemporary history.

Source. "Federal Data Protection Act (BDSG), In the version promulgated on 14 January 2003 (Federal Law Gazette I, p. 66), last amended by Article 1 of the Act of 14 August 2009 (Federal Law Gazette I, p. 2814)"

In addition to anonymization also storage and Informed Consent principles are mentioned.

Chapter 10, Legal Requirements & Regulations provides more details in this context.

2.4 Biobanks – What do we Mean by That?

There are numerous definitions of biobanks, all differing in the scope of the material to be stored, the protection masks applied, and the population collected samples come from.

The Public Population Project in Genomics (P3G) defines a biobank/biorepository in its Population Biobanks Lexicon of July 2007 as

> *"An organized collection of human biological material and associated information stored for one or more research purposes." (cf. (9))*

The Biobanks Act of Sweden, promulgated on 23 May 2002, defines the term biobank as

> *"biological material from one or more human beings that is collected and preserved for an indefinite or limited period and, whose origin is traceable to an individual or individuals."*

Anonymized samples are not covered by this definition.

According to the German National Ethics Council (Nationaler Ethikrat) Opinion on Biobanks for research, 2004,

> *Biobanks are "collections of samples of human bodily substances (e.g. cells, tissue, blood, or DNA as the physical medium of genetic information) that are or can be associated with personal data and information on their donors."*

We will provide and use a slightly different definition of biobanks in clinical research. In our understanding:

> *Biobanks used in clinical research are "collections of anonymized samples of human bodily substances" (e.g. cells, tissue, blood, or DNA as the physical medium of genetic information) that can be associated with data and information on their donors, whereas the data related to the donor are held separately. Supplementary data to the sample and hence to genetic data derived therefrom can be merged on request, but a trace back to the donors' identity is not possible due to anonymization."*

An overview of legal and ethical issues arising in the context of biobanking in Europe is given in (10), "Outstanding legal and ethical issues on biobanks, *An overview on the regulations of member states of the EuroBioBank project*".

In order to avoid confusions it is strongly recommended to clearly define what type of biobank is being considered prior to starting any discussion on this topic.

3 Protection Masks and Procedures

Most of the contradictions and misunderstandings in the context of handling genetic data result from the confounding of distinct terms used in this area.

As an example, the study mode used and the degree of protection (the so-called **protection mask**) provided to data and samples on the one hand, and the methods that are used to realize these protection masks on the other hand, must be clearly distinguished, but are often mixed in reality.

That is why the first step of our approach consists in unambiguously defining the different kinds of protection masks as well as the methods needed for their implementation. A good survey of terms used, is given in (8), and (11).

We basically follow the definitions of the EMA (cf. (7)) with respect to the introduced categories for samples and data, with some enhancements providing clarification where it seems to be adequate.

There are only 3 different protection masks for data and samples, i.e. samples/data can be:
- *Identified*
- *De-identified*
- *Anonymized*

We will explain the fundamentals of these protection masks in the following.

3.1 Identified Samples/Data

Identified samples/data are samples/data that are labeled with the name of the subject the samples/data come from, or in another unique way giving the identity of the respective subject (Fig. 3.1). In this sense, a PAT_NO (Patient Number) does not allow to identify a subject in one step, whereas the use of a social security number as a unique identifier provides the same low level of protection to privacy as the subject's name itself.
- The process of providing identified data is called **identification.**
- The result of an identification process are **identified data** and/or **identified samples.**

Identification can be realized by different methods, e.g.
- Identification by name.
- Identification by initials.
- Identification by the social security number.

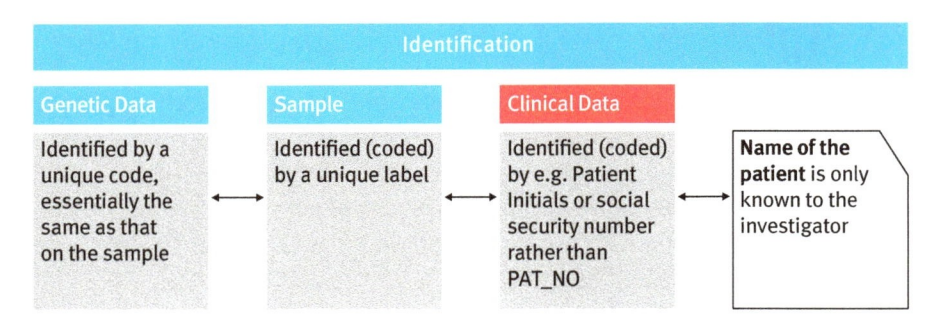

Identification		
Genetic Data	**Sample**	**Clinical Data**
Identified by a unique code, essentially the same as that on the sample	Identified (coded) by a unique label	Identified (coded) by e.g. Patient Initials or social security number rather than PAT_NO

Name of the patient is only known to the investigator

Fig. 3.1 Data Identification

3.2 De-identified Samples/Data

De-identified samples/data are samples/data that are labeled with a code rather than the name of the subject the samples/data come from. A trace back to the individual subject is still possible, but only the investigator can relate a PAT_NO to the patient's name.

Clinical data identified by a TRI_NO (Trial Number) and PAT_NO (Patient Number) are considered being de-identified data.

De-identification can be implemented in several ways, dependent on the protection level required.
- The process of providing de-identified data/samples is called **de-identification**
- The result of a de-identification process are **de-identified data** and/or **de-identified samples**

3.3 Anonymized Samples/Data

Anonymized samples/data are samples/data that are labeled with a code rather than the name of a subject, **and** a trace back to the individual subject is no longer possible.
- Anonymization is the process of breaking the relationship between the subjects' identity on the one hand and the respective clinical data and related samples on the other hand and simultaneously retaining the relationship between the clinical data and the related samples
- The result of an anonymization process are **anonymized data** and/or **anonymized samples**

It will be explained later how anonymization of clinical data and samples is reached.
Anonymization can be performed at two stages
- **Immediate anonymization (pre-genetic evaluation anonymization)**,

i.e., anonymization prior to evaluating genetic data; this is a must when applying unspecified mode.
- **Deferred anonymization (post-genetic evaluation anonymization)**,
  i.e., anonymization after evaluating genetic data.

In this case, the anonymization process gets as input samples/data having an original protection mask identified or de-identified, i.e. samples/data that have been stored either as identified or de-identified samples/data for a certain time.

3.4 Re-identification

The process of tracing back from de-identified samples/data to the individual subject is called re-identification.
- **Re-identification** is only possible for de-identified samples/data.
- **Anonymized** samples/data do not allow a re-identification.

Anonymized samples/data provide the highest level of privacy protection by precluding the identification of individuals.

4 Coding Methods for De-identified Samples/Data

De-identification can be realized by different methods. Two methods of providing de-identified samples/data are currently in use:
- **De-identification** by **single coding** (e.g., PAT_NO, single random code).
- **De-identification** by **double coding** (label exchange).

The protection level of samples/data can be augmented if for instance de-identification is implemented by a **triple coding** (twofold label exchange) process. (cf. details below)

4.1 Single-coded Samples/Data

Single-coded samples/data are those samples/data having a random code as identifier instead of the individual's name (Fig. 4.1). Only the investigator knows the identity (the name) of the individual to whom the respective code applies, and
- the investigator usually holds the key to the code.

The PAT_NO (patient number) is usually considered to be such a code. This may be sufficient when only clinical data are included in a subsequent evaluation, but whenever genetic data are involved, the protection level is low compared to those records identified by a randomly generated code. This is mainly due to the applied allocation methods for PAT_NOs.

In multicenter clinical trials, a range of possible PAT_NOs is allocated to every center. So if 100 patients are planned for center no. 1, we could provide PAT_NOs in the range of 100 to 200 for that center. PAT_NOs in that center are usually assigned according to the sequence of entering the trial. The medication number itself is randomly assigned. The ranges of PAT_NOs reserved for respective centers is known to the sponsor. That is why the patient's identity is slightly revealed, if the number of treated patients within a center is very small, e.g. less than 10 (Fig. 4.2).

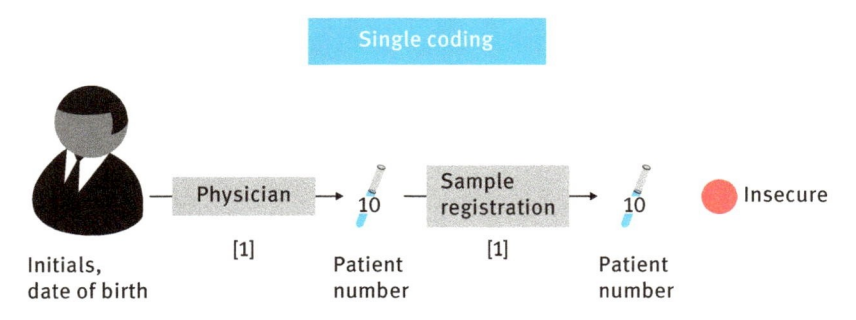

Fig. 4.1. Single Coding

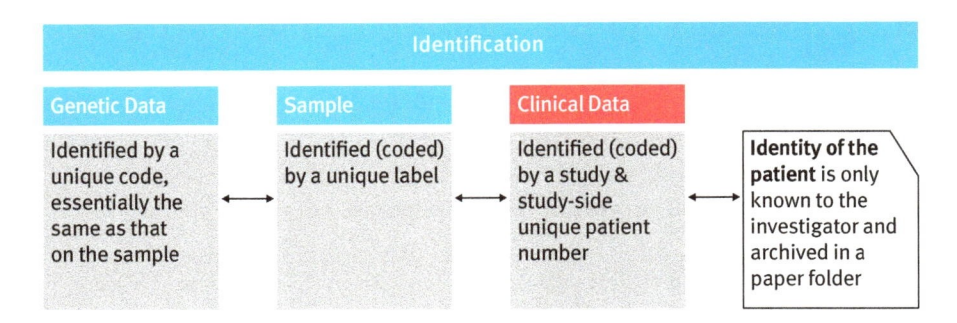

Fig. 4.2 Single Coding Procedure

Nevertheless, this allocation method produces single-coded samples/data according to the definition given above, although the protection decreases with an increasing number of centers involved (only few patients per center).

4.2 Double-coded Samples/Data

Double-coded samples/data are those samples/data having at the outset a first random code as identifier instead of the individual's name (Fig. 4.3). Only the investigator knows the identity (the name) of the individual to whom the respective code applies, and
– the investigator usually holds the key to the first code.

In a second step, the first code on the samples is exchanged, e.g. by a central logistic CRO or by the staff of a biobank prior to storing the samples.
– The key to the second code is held by a central, secured protection database.

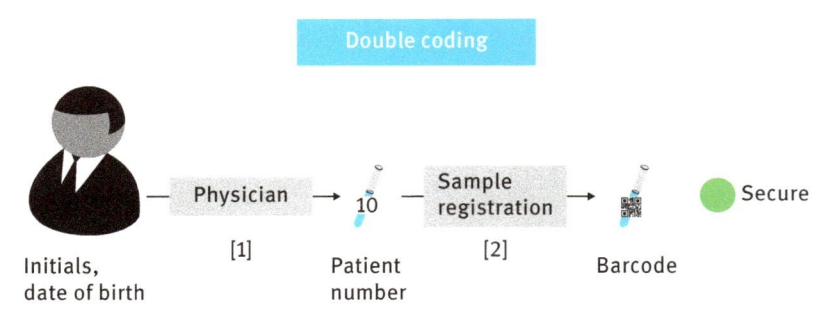

Fig. 4.3 Double Coding

Neither the knowledge of the first code nor the knowledge of the second code is sufficient to trace back to the individual's identity. The knowledge of both codes and their mutual link are necessary to re-identify an individual (patient).

Anyone with knowledge of the pharmacogenetic results can only trace a subject identity to a coded identifier but no further (Fig. 4.4).

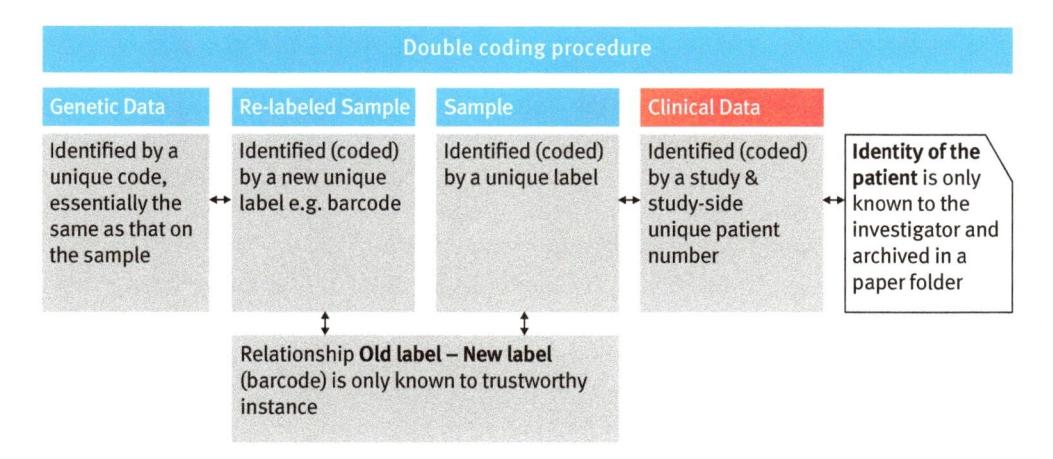

Double coding procedure				
Genetic Data	**Re-labeled Sample**	**Sample**	**Clinical Data**	
Identified by a unique code, essentially the same as that on the sample	Identified (coded) by a new unique label e.g. barcode	Identified (coded) by a unique label	Identified (coded) by a study & study-side unique patient number	**Identity of the patient** is only known to the investigator and archived in a paper folder
	Relationship **Old label – New label** (barcode) is only known to trustworthy instance			

Fig. 4.4 Double Coding Procedure

The **EMA** (cf. (6)) provides some recommendations as to where to hold the key for the second coding:

> The key to the double code might be maintained by the sponsoring organization, in areas entrusted with maintaining confidential information (e.g. legal, quality assurance, clinical statistics) under strict operating procedures.
> Alternatively, the key might be held by an external entity, such as governmental agency, legal counsel, or other qualified third party not involved with the research.

4.3 Triple-coded Samples/Data

Triple-coded samples/data are quite similar to double-coded samples/data described above (Fig. 4.5) . Triple coded samples/data at the outset have a first random code (Patient ID) as identifier instead of the individual's name and a random barcode 1. A blood sample is identified by both identifiers. Only the investigator knows the identity (the name) of the individual to whom the respective code applies, and
– the investigator usually holds the key to the first code.

In a second step, the first code (Patient ID) and barcode 1 are registered prior to removing the Patient-ID from the sample. Only barcode 1 remains on the sample. This can be done e.g. by a central logistic CRO or by the staff of a biobank prior to storing the samples.
– The Patient ID and barcode 1 are held by a central, secured protection database.

In the third step, executed by a different staff with the logistic CRO, barcode 1 is replaced by a random barcode 2, the final identifier of samples and data.
– Barcode 2 is also held by a central, secured protection database.

The triple coding process is called factual anonymization. It is more personnel-intensive than any other coding process but ensures a security like anonymization with all the advantages of pseudonymization.

No one in the process chain gets any access to both identifiers (Patient ID and barcode 2) neither technically nor organizationally.

Neither the knowledge of the first or second code nor the knowledge of the third code is sufficient to trace back to the individuals identity. The knowledge of both codes and their mutual link are necessary to re-identify an individual (patient).

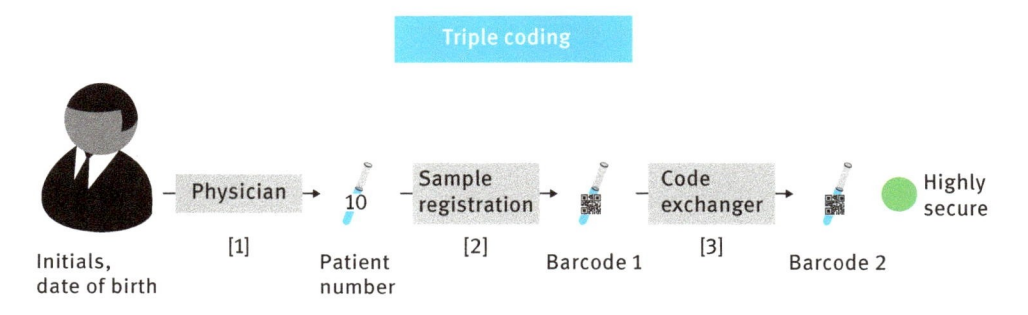

Fig. 4.5 Triple Coding

5 Relationships Among the Protection Masks

The diagram in Fig. 5.1 reflects the relationships among the 3 possible protection masks

Protection mask – Summary

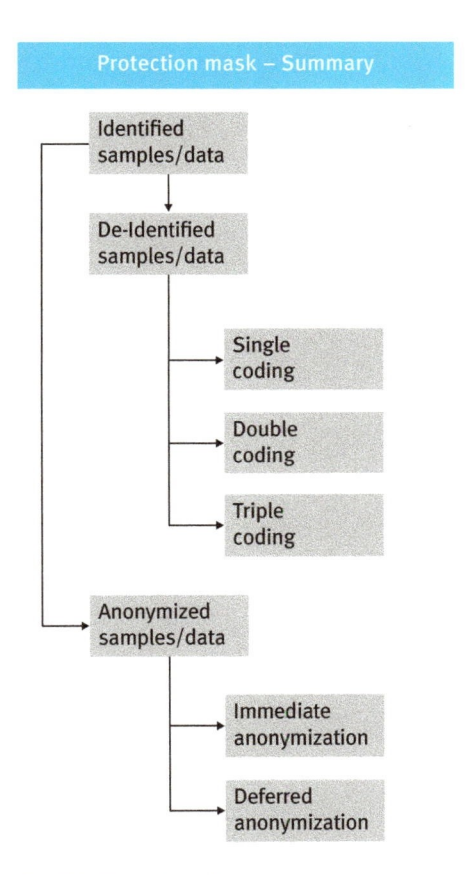

- Identified samples/data
  - De-Identified samples/data
    - Single coding
    - Double coding
    - Triple coding
  - Anonymized samples/data
    - Immediate anonymization
    - Deferred anonymization

Fig. 5.1 Protection Masks

6 Data Types

Do you really know how to define **personal** data? Well, here are two examples.
Which of these can be said to provide personal data?
- (Obama, US, male, Washington,......)
- (123, F, female, Paris,....)

The first idea will certainly be "example No 1, these are personal data", because the record contains the name of a person.

Identifying Data	
(Name of a person, data ...)	Identity is known,
(Social security number, data ...)	personal data
(Patients initials, data ...)	identified

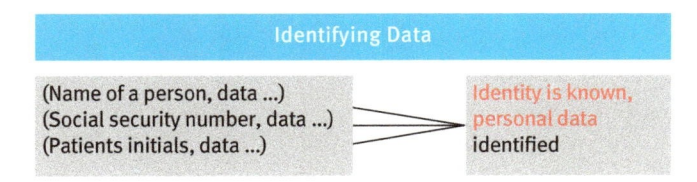

Fig. 6.1 Identifying Data

That's correct, strictly speaking, the first record provides identified personal data. But the second record also provides personal data, without directly revealing the identity of their owner.

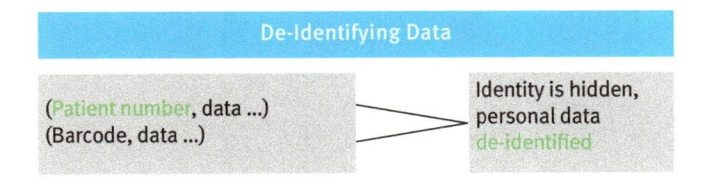

De-Identifying Data	
(Patient number, data ...)	Identity is hidden,
(Barcode, data ...)	personal data
	de-identified

Fig. 6.2 De-Identifying Data

Strictly speaking, the second record provides de-identified personal data. The identification of the record – the identifying key – is accomplished by a code "123" rather than a name. The identity of the owner is hidden, but as long as somebody knows the identity of the owner, i.e. as long as somebody can trace back to the owner's identity the data provided by record 2 are personal data.

If a trace back to the person's identity is always possible we speak of personal data (Fig. 6.3).

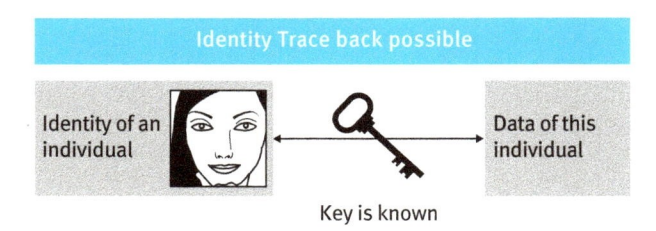

Fig. 6.3 Possible Identity Trace Back

A trace back to the person's identity is not possible under any circumstances – then we do not speak of personal data (Fig. 6.4).

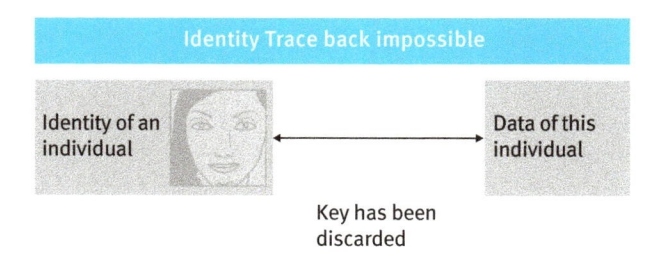

Fig. 6.4 Impossible Identity Trace Back

When conducting clinical studies we are working with personal data (Fig. 6.5).

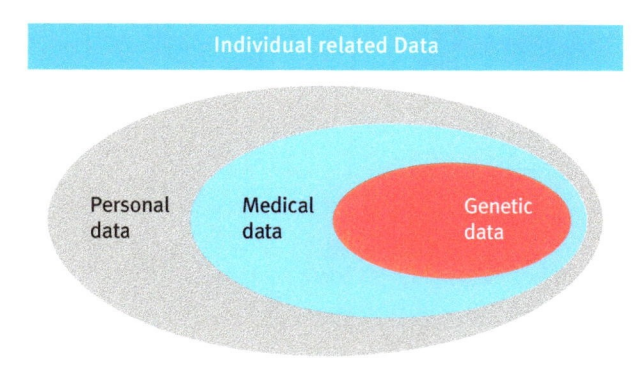

Fig. 6.5 Individual Related Data

and essentially with a subset of personal data, with medical data. Whenever a clinical study is supplemented with a collection of material used to extract DNA of the subjects involved in that study, we are not only working with medical data but also with a subset of those data, genetic data.

Is there any reliable source where these data types have been clearly defined? Indeed, we can find respective definitions for one or several of the abovementioned data types in the data protection laws of every country.

The German Federal Data Protection Act defines Personal data as follows:

Federal Data Protection Act (Germany), Section 3, Further Definitions
(1) **Personal data** means any information concerning the personal or material circumstances of an identified or identifiable individual (the data subject).

We will not find definitions for medical and genetic data there, and even the EU Privacy Directive does not provide definitions for medical and genetic data.

However, "the Appendix to Recommendation No. R (97) 5 of the Committee of Ministers to Member States on the Protection of Medical Data" (cf. (43) or 16.2)) provides clear definitions of all three data types.

7 Anonymization

7.1 Basic Terms and Ideas

What does anonymization mean?

Anonymization is the process of breaking the relationship between the patient's (subject's) identity on the one hand and the respective clinical data and related samples on the other hand and simultaneously retaining the relationship between the clinical data and the related samples.

The procedures and measures to be applied must guarantee that a trace back to the subject's identity is no longer possible after anonymization (Fig. 7.1). This also implies that:
- After anonymization there is no possibility to correct or enhance clinical data, to supplement sample information, or to identify samples; i.e. all information necessary for the usage of samples – storage time, restrictions made by Ethics Committees in general – must be attached to the samples prior to anonymization, in order not to get lost when conducting the anonymization process.
- A withdrawal and a destruction of samples after anonymization are not possible.

What are the prerequisites for anonymization?

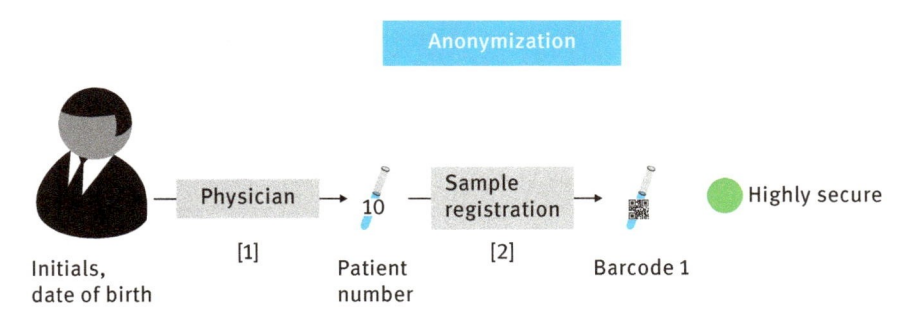

Fig. 7.1 Anonymization

The anonymization process consists of three fundamental steps that must be taken into account:
- Masking of attributes that could reveal the subject's identity.
- Discarding the identifying key without losing the relationship between anonymized clinical data and respective genetic samples. This measure is necessary in order to prevent anybody from tracing back to the subject's identity.
- Implementing security measures to prevent a breach of anonymization by simply matching anonymized and respective non anonymized data.

Bear in mind that anonymization is an irreversible process that does not allow a trace back to the subject's identity, that is why all tasks requiring the knowledge of the identifying key must be done prior to the invocation of the anonymization process. We will go into more details when presenting the general framework for anonymization.

Tab. 7.1 Study Modes – Protection Masks – Technical & Organizational Realization

Study Mode	Prespecified	Unspecified
Protection Mask of Data & Samples	De-identified	Anonymized
Technical & Organizational Realization	Single Coding Double Coding Triple Coding	– Key Exchange – Masking of Variables – Prevent Matching of de-identified and respective anonymized Data

7.2 Masking

An important aspect of the anonymization process is the so-called masking of variables that could reveal the subject's identity, even if the key to the subject's identity has been discarded.

Masking of a variable is the process of replacing the original content of that variable by another reasonable content without changing the format of the variable. This does not mean that the content of a variable must be always replaced throughout; it is often sufficient and also meaningful to replace only the critical values of a variable by another reasonable content, so that patient's privacy can be guaranteed furthermore.

Changing the format of a variable, e.g. replacing a date by the respective year would prevent you from reusing existing statistical evaluation programs, i.e.
– Variable formats must be retained, to allow statistical analysis with existing programs (e.g. check for shift in population).

> **Context sensitive Data De-Identification – Sample I**
>
> (Random number, profession, date of birth ...)
> (12345432986516, physician, 1960/03/29 ...)

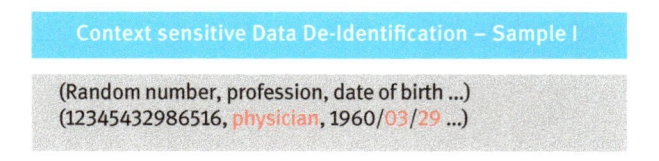

Fig. 7.2 Context Sensitive De-Identification I

The example in Fig. 7.2 provides a record with non-personal data, the identity of the subject is not known under any circumstances.

The content "physician" does not reveal the subject's identity, because the profession physician does not allow to uniquely identify the owner of that record.

The example in Fig. 7.3 provides a record that is quite similar to the first. Both records have the same structure, but the second record differs slightly in the content of the field "profession".

Context sensitive Data De-Identification – Sample II

(Random number, profession, date of birth ...)
(12345432986516, data protection officer of Germany, ...)

Fig. 7.3 Context Sensitive De-Identification II

Whereas the identity of the subject related to the first record is by no means revealed by its profession "physician", the identity of the second subject is no longer hidden. Data protection officer of Germany is a unique position at any time; i.e. the identity of the subject owning this record is known, at least indirectly, so the record displays personal data.

Is there nevertheless a way to guarantee anonymity of the data? Well, that can only be reached by slightly modifying the critical content of variables concerned so that an identification based on those fields is no longer possible, i.e. the critical content of fields must be modified so that the identity of the record owner remains hidden.

Context sensitive Data De-Identification – Sample III

(Random number, profession, date of birth ...)
(12345432986516, ABCDFGS, 1960/06/30, ...)

Fig. 7.4 Context Sensitive De-Identification III

In our example above we could hide the identity of the record owner by replacing the content of the field profession by an arbitrary content, if adequate, and the exact date of birth in general by a date adjusted to the mid of the respective year, i.e. replace the record of Fig. 7.2 by the record of Fig. 7.4. Masking of variables is related to a certain loss of information, that is why we should carefully check the question:

Is masking really necessary?
Yes it is, there are groups of variables that could directly reveal the identity of a data subject, even if the identifying key has been discarded, i.e. replaced by a random number. Those variables that might immediately reflect the identity of a data subject must be always masked.

Which variables are concerned?
As a first approach we direct your attention to the Health Insurance Portability and Accountability Act (HIPAA) Privacy Rules (cf. (12), (13), (14)). According to the proposals made there, the following variables, if ever collected, should be checked for the necessity of a masking process:
- Names.
- All geographic subdivisions smaller than a state.
- All elements of dates (except year) concerning dates directly related to the data subject, including birth date, admission date, discharge date, date of death; and all ages over 89 and all elements of dates (including year) indicative of such age, except that such ages and elements may be aggregated into a single category of age '90 or older'.
- Medical record numbers.

Bear in mind that some variables as specified by the HIPAA Privacy Rules, e.g. patient data like initials or addresses are never collected in the context of conducting clinical trials!

You should carefully check each variable used within a clinical study for the necessity of masking.

The following clinical variables are candidates for masking:
- Dates related to special examinations like physical examination, laboratory/pharmacogenetic sampling-, and questionnaire date.
- Informed consent dates: informed consent date for participation in a clinical study, informed consent date for genetic analysis.
- Date of randomization.
- Dates related to trial drugs, i.e. dispension date, date of first and last intake, most recent intake dates, date when medication code has been broken, etc.
- Dates related to adverse events and concomitant therapies, i.e. start dates, end dates.
- Trial termination date.

As mentioned above, masking is always associated with a certain loss of information. Some variables must be always masked, independent of the specific statistical evaluations, e.g. special dates. Other variables require only a context sensitive masking, i.e. a masking on a per analysis basis. It is therefore recommended to implement masking as a two-step procedure:
- **Masking prior to Anonymization**
  The original content of the respective variables is lost for all further statistical analyses.

- **Context Sensitive Masking**
  The decision whether a variable must be masked is often highly dependent on the data to be included in the respective statistical analysis, masking in such a situation is associated with a temporary loss of information only.

Often the information provided by only one variable is so striking that it is sufficient to uniquely identify the related subject.

In general, extreme values of variables are critical values that could implicitly reveal the identity of the subject related to that data. Examples could be an age above 90 years, a weight over 200 kg or an extremely high blood pressure of a person suffering from hypertension.

It would make no sense to mask those variables prior to anonymization, i.e. once for all; the loss of information would be tremendous. But, how could we escape from this situation? Well, aggregation or truncation are the appropriate measures to be applied. Aggregate the extreme values of concerned variables on a per analysis basis. The original content of the respective variables is lost only temporarily; i.e. lost for the specified statistical analysis only.

Height and weight are variables that are always collected in a clinical study as a standard part of patient's demographics. Extreme values of both variables could normally enable us to trace back to the subject's identity. It is therefore necessary to aggregate extreme values into one category, e.g. all weights over 90 kg could be combined into one weight class *"over 90 kg"*, and all heights over 185 cm could be also combined into one height class *"over 185 cm"*. In order not to lose the original format of these variables, you have to replace all weight values greater or equal to 90 by the value 90, and all height values greater or equal to 185 by the value 185.

But is it really necessary to mask weight and height in each study? No, even if a bit surprising, it actually isn't always necessary. Imagine you have set up a clinical trial, where one inclusion criteria is *"overweight"*, e.g. weight over 100 kg. In such a clinical study a weight of 110 kg would be by no means an extreme value. This implies:

The decision whether a specific value of a collected variable is to be considered as an extreme value depends on the context in which this variable has been collected and also on the context in which this specific variable will be analyzed. We call such a characteristic of a variable **"context sensitive"**.

7.2.1 A Way to Detect Variables to be Masked

Prior to starting the masking process you should answer the following questions:
- Which variables must be masked?
- When has masking to be done – prior to anonymization and/or context sensitive?
- How should masking be done – is a format reserving algorithm for the replacement of specific values of variables already available?

As outlined already, whereas some variables must be always masked, there are other variables that require a context sensitive masking decision, i.e. whether or not a variable has to be masked often depends on the data which are delivered for the statistical evaluation. Variables to be masked context sensitively have to be determined on a per request for a common statistical analysis of anonymized clinical and related genetic data basis.

How to proceed in practice?
The first step is always the identification of variables that could have critical values requiring most likely a masking procedure.
For instance, those variables are dates, names, positions, and in general special grouping variables.
A way to go, we recommend with emphasis, is the distinction between static – and dynamic variables, whereby
- **static variables** are variables that do not change their values over time. These category of variables is more critical than
- **dynamic variables,** which have time dependent values, i.e. values that may vary with time.

The height of adults, e.g. subjects with an age over 30, is independent of time, whereas the height of children varies with time, i.e. it is increasing with time. Within the adult group height is a static variable, whereas within the children group height is a dynamic variable.
- Variables that may change the category (static – dynamic) dependent on the subject the respective values have been collected from, are called **conditioned static variables**

Weight of a data subject is time dependent and thus a dynamic variable. But bear in mind, this does not mean that weight would be uncritical, extreme values must be aggregated or categorized, as outlined above, prior to any statistical analysis.
A genetic pattern or a special genotype are examples for static variables that do not change their values over time. A genetic pattern represents in a certain sense a fingerprint that could directly identify a subject. That is why those data are highly sensitive and require therefore itemized and sophisticated rules to protect the privacy of the data subject related.
We can fix as a rule of thumb:
- Static variables are more critical than conditioned static or dynamic variables.

In a second step we must identify those variables that are critical, independent of their special values. These variables must always undergo the masking procedure, i.e.

- the masking rules must be applied to all values of those variables and not only to the extremes.

The second step, i.e. the detection of critical variables that are always subjected to a masking procedure must be performed prior to anonymization.

After anonymization but prior to the start of any statistical evaluation of anonymized clinical and related genetic data we must check whether context sensitive masking is adequate.

The necessity of context sensitive masking is primarily dependent on the data to be requested for analysis. A too small number of subjects per center may be critical with respect to privacy protection of the data subjects on the one hand, i.e. center number would be critical in this special case and must be preferably masked. On the other hand, the knowledge of the center number will be of great worth if differences in results are conjectured to be basically related to differences in the specific trial handling of centers. This implies that center number is a candidate for context sensitive masking rather than masking throughout, although center number is a static variable.
- In oncology studies the date of death is often used as a primary endpoint and needed for survival data analysis purposes, e.g. Kaplan-Meier analysis. Although we have recognized dates as critical variables, the particular worth of "*date of death*" is highly dependent on the study design. In an oncology study this variable is of major value, whereas in CNS study date of death might be of minor value only, i.e. not specified as primary endpoint.

These examples show that we must carefully check which variables have to undergo a masking procedure prior to anonymization, i.e. which variables must be masked throughout, and which variables are candidates for context sensitive masking in the first instance (Fig. 7.5). Bear in mind:

Information once lost is lost forever and cannot be rebuilt.

Masking is a highly responsible task requiring a deep knowledge of statistical methods to be applied. If we don't know the worth of specific variables we might release variables for the primary masking process, which are of tremendous worth.

Masking is also a highly responsible task requiring a deep knowledge of laws and regulations that must be met in the context of privacy protection.

This implies that we should involve experienced biostatistician(s) and experienced data protection experts in the agreement upon masking rules to be applied.

Masking of Data		
Time of masking	**Variables to be included**	**Loss of information**
Prior to... — Part of the Anonymization process, one time execution	Variables to be masked throughout, e.g. PAT_No ✓ Static variables ✓ Conditioned static variables ✓ Dynamic variables	High ↓ Low — Variable content lost once for all
Anonymization – Anonymization – Anonymization – Anonymization – Anonymization		
After... — Context sensitive, request, subrequest based, on demand execution	✓ Static variables ✓ Conditioned static variables ✓ Dynamic variables	High ↓ Low — Variable content only temporarily lost

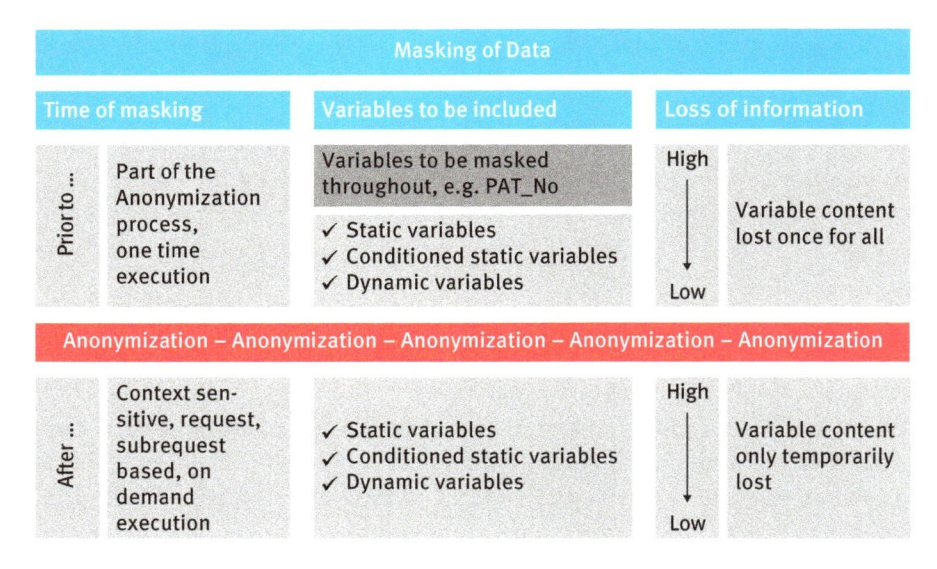

Fig. 7.5 Masking of Data

7.3 Discarding the Key

7.3.1 From Sample Collection to Sample Registration

The anonymization process involves three independent entities:
- The **clinical data** to be anonymized.
- The **samples** to be labeled with randomized unique barcodes.
- The **key relationship** between clinical data and samples.

Upon collection
The clinical data (clinical records) are usually identified by a trial number, a patient number, and, if necessary, by some supplementary attributes.
   We call this identifying key
- **C**linical **D**ata **I**dentifier (**CDI**)

Upon collection, samples for a future common statistical analysis of anonymized clinical and related genetic data are identified by a
- **G**enetic **D**ata **I**dentifier (**GDI**)

The relationship between clinical data and related samples is known. At this stage of a clinical study CDI and GDI are even identical in most cases. In the course of the whole sample handling process none of the identifiers will change prior to sample registration, and

Sample registration is the process of registering samples, collected from patients participating in a clinical study

Upon sample registration
- The GDI label attached to the sample is replaced by a unique barcode, the **nGDI** (**n**ew **G**enetic **D**ata **I**dentifier), and the clinical record identifier (CDI) is retained. Replacement of the old label means to remove the old label and attach a new one (barcode) to the respective sample.
- The initial key relationship between clinical data and samples, CDI – GDI, is replaced by the new key relationship CDI – nGDI and stored securely and separately from data and samples in a protected database – the anonymized – or de-identified **K**ey **P**rotection **D**ata**B**ase (**KPDB**), dependent on whether samples are registered for anonymized or de-identified genetic analysis.
- After registration, samples are identified by the barcode nGDI and neither sample records nor data records to be derived later contain any pointer to the related clinical data.

Replacing the old label by a new barcode increases the privacy protection level of the registered samples. The **K**ey **P**rotection **D**ata**B**ase is the instance that exclusively knows the relationship between patient number and respective samples.

7.3.2 Ethical Committee Restrictions

From a legal point of view there should be no objections that could be raised with respect to a genetic analysis based on anonymized clinical data and related samples. Nevertheless, Ethics Committees may raise such objections restricting the analysis to be performed in the future. In any case, we must guarantee that collected samples are only used for the purpose granted by the donor through a genetic informed consent, taking into account all restrictions made by Ethics Committees, Institutional Review Boards (IRBs), etc.

What does this mean in practice?
Well, this simply means: upon registration of a sample we are obliged to attach all information regarding the use of the respective sample to that sample, i.e. all supplementary information describing the possible use of a sample must be attached to that sample prior to the start of the anonymization process.

Be aware that there will be no possibility to trace back to the subject's identity after having successfully passed an anonymization procedure.

Which objections could be raised by Ethics Committees, resp. IRBs?
- Limitations of storage duration of samples and genetic test results is sometimes required on a per study site basis.

Agreeing upon a common start date for storage is a realistic approach, specify e.g. storage of samples for "*at most x years*" after dblock (lock of the clinical database). Do not specify "*for at least x years*", this would mean "*no restrictions*" at all. The start of a common analysis of anonymized clinical and related genetic data is always after anonymization, and anonymization will never be performed prior to dblock. The collection times of individual samples within a large clinical study may be spread over several years, that is why a storage duration management based on individual samples is hard to realize and does not make much sense, too.

Another objection Ethics Committees, resp. IRBs may raise is
- the restriction of the planned genetic analysis to the therapeutic area(s) the test drugs are designed for.

In this special case released therapeutic area(s) must be attached to the individual samples, so that all samples authorized for the planned analysis can be easily identified upon request for a common analysis of anonymized clinical and related genetic samples/data. The restriction to therapeutic area(s) is a restriction on a per study site basis, settled by an Ethic Committee resp. IRB for all study sites in its area of responsibility.

Sometimes Ethics Committees resp. IRBs raise even more restrictive objections, i.e.
- restrictions not only to therapeutic area(s) but also to individual indications.

If more than one indication is handled within one clinical trial – e.g. different tumor categories within an oncology trial – then the required restrictions are no longer center related but patient related and must be therefore stored on a per patient basis in the clinical database. Ethical Committee Restrictions are clinical data, resp. clinical meta data, and by no means part of the administrative data of a clinical study, usually stored in a clinical trial management system.

Bear in mind that statisticians involved in the common evaluation of anonymized clinical and related genetic data are not aware of the individual restrictions attached to samples; they only get the samples and/or data of those data subjects where attached restrictions and required analysis are in balance, i.e. where area(s) of evaluation are covered by the attached (stored) area(s) of restrictions.

The trial number itself is needed and must be retained to later on enable us to select samples belonging to comparable trials, i.e. we do not advice to replace the trial number by a random number. This decision is by no means counterproductive to anonymization. Checking the structure of clinical data would unambiguously reveal which trials are being included in an analysis. That is why a masking of the trial number would not result in an additional data protection effect.

Remember, our goal is to protect the patient's privacy, and this goal is reached by implementing the proposed anonymization process. Moreover, trial numbers can be hidden to the evaluating staff by applying context sensitive masking, if adequate.

7.3.3 The Last Check Prior to Discarding the Key

Immediately prior to the start of the anonymization procedure
Check whether
- agreed masking rules are available, so that the anonymization algorithm can mask the respective variables accordingly when invoked.
- clinical data are complete and consistent.
- informed consents are complete and consistent.
- registration of samples is complete and consistent.
- all withdrawal requests have been solved.

Remember, the anonymization process must not be invoked, if
- clinical data are incomplete and/or inconsistent, or
- if any informed consent information is missing or unclear, or
- if the registration of samples relating to patients of the respective study is not yet complete, or
- if there are any non-confirmed withdrawal requests.

It is recommended to clear open questions in the context of Informed Consent (IC) check as soon as possible, i.e. we strongly recommend to permanently check
- whether all samples, already registered, have a positive IC, and
- whether samples have already been registered for every available positive IC.

Start the anonymization process if and only if all relevant issues have been solved satisfactorily, i.e. prior to the start of the anonymization process prove that all legal requirements are met.

Remember, anonymization is an irreversible process.

7.3.4 What Happens When "Discarding the Key"?

Upon start of the anonymization algorithm:
- Clinical data to be anonymized are identified by a CDI.

- Related samples are identified by a nGDI (GDI has been replaced by nGDI upon sample registration), and
- the relationship between CDI and nGDI is exclusively and securely stored in the key protection database (KPDB).

The anonymization algorithm replaces simultaneously the identifying key CDI in the clinical data to be anonymized as well as in the key relation CDI – nGDI of the key protection database by a new identifying key, the
- **n**ew **C**linical **D**ata **I**dentifier (**nCDI**).

Having finished the anonymization algorithm:
- Clinical data are anonymized and identified by the new key nCDI. The anonymized clinical data do not contain any pointer to the related samples, or to the genetic data derived later on.
- Samples are also anonymized and still identified by nGDI, and do not contain any pointer to the related anonymized clinical data, and
- the new key relationship nCDI – nGDI is exclusively and securely stored in the key protection database (KPDB). The KPDB is the only entity that knows how anonymized clinical data and samples/genetic data are related.

What does this actually mean?
The applied anonymization model, i.e. the realization of a strict separation of the three entities *anonymized clinical data*, *samples/genetic data*, and *key relationship* implements an additional level of data protection.

Nobody is able to merge anonymized clinical data and respective genetic data, derived from the related samples, without the explicit support of the key protection database, even if he/she had access to both data sources (Fig. 7.6).

The *three entities approach*, referred to as the SDK (**S**ample, **D**ata, **K**ey) approach, induces in a natural way how a common analysis of anonymized clinical and related genetic data must be performed, i.e. the necessary merging of both data sources can only, namely exclusively, be performed on request by the **K**ey **P**rotection **D**ata**B**ase. That is why
- The key relationship nCDI – nGDI will never leave the **K**ey **P**rotection **D**ata**B**ase KPDB.

An itemized description of how such a request management must be set up and how the key relationship nCDI – nGDI can be retained, will be given later in chapter 9 *Request Management*.

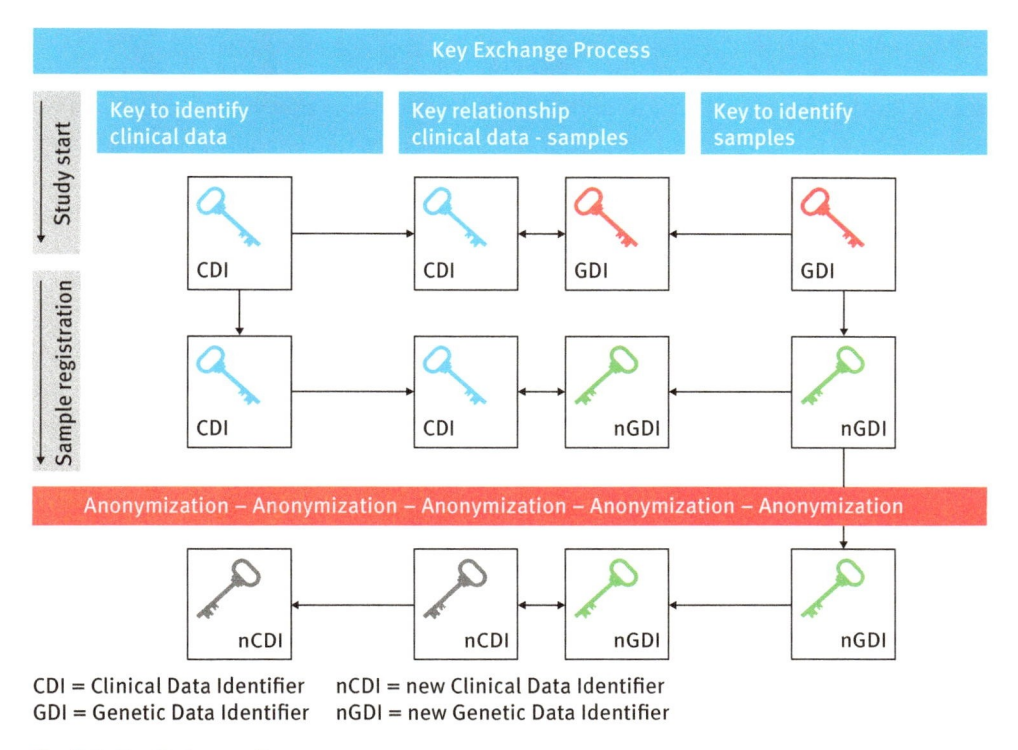

Fig. 7.6 Key Exchange Process

CDI = Clinical Data Identifier
GDI = Genetic Data Identifier
nCDI = new Clinical Data Identifier
nGDI = new Genetic Data Identifier

To avoid an unauthorized access to key relationships when anonymization is pending, it is strongly recommended to encrypt the respective key values by means of Advanced Encryption Standard (AES).

The special key needed for encryption should be created and held securely by the application server used.

7.4 Maintaining the Reliability of Stored Data

When working with data, not only clinical and/or genetic data, you must guarantee that data used are free of logical contradictions. What does this mean? Well, during data entry, collected data are mostly either already available in a coded form or are being coded as part of the overall data entry process. The applied coding methods are on the one hand company or hospital internal coding standards and on the other hand internationally agreed coding standards of medicine like
- MedDRA, – **Med**ical **D**ictionary for **R**egulatory **A**ctivities
- SNOMED, SNOMED CT, – **S**ystematized **No**menclature of **Med**icine – **C**linical **T**erms
- WHO-DD – **WHO D**rug **D**ictionary

Company or hospital internal coding standards are for example codes for gender or codes for ordinal scales, used to monitor pain and efficacy. There will arise no problems as long as the classification of the applied scales does not change, i.e. no objections can be raised as long as you apply the same scale throughout. When changing the classification of a scale, e.g. when applying a five point pain scale instead of a four point pain scale, the related pain variable must be changed, too. Nevertheless, these facts are often ignored.

A variable MP (**M**orning **P**ain) recorded on a four point pain scale is not the same as a variable MP measured on a five point pain scale. Different pain scales require also different variables' names. Use MP4 and MP5 instead of MP only. Variables having the same name, but being measured differently, must not be combined in an overall analysis. These problems can be easily resolved by implementing respective organizational measures.

Another more sophisticated problem usually arises in the context of internationally agreed coding standards in medicine and genetics.

When using internationally agreed coding systems with clinical and genetic data, which is the standard, you should take care that within one trial always the same coding system and the same version of the applied coding system is used. This is especially important in multinational studies.

In general, the coding systems are updated on a yearly basis. As long as data are stored and no longer used there will arise no problems. Selecting data from different trials being coded with different versions of the same coding systems may cause problems because the code of the same topic may have changed. Often a coded category is split into several new categories and consequently coded in a different manner. In any case, prior to starting a common statistical evaluation of anonymized clinical and related genetic data, you must ensure that:

- All data in the anonymized database have the same coding standard, i.e. the same coding system and the same version of the respective coding system must be used throughout.
- An update strategy for respective coded variables is available upon import of data.

Two strategies are conceivable to adjust the coding to the necessary actual standard:
- Updating immediately after publication of new coding versions,

or
- Updating prior to the start of the common statistical evaluation of anonymized clinical and related genetic data.

Updating prior to statistical analysis implies that you must store the coding system used, the respective version upon coding and all available new versions and update files together with the clinical data concerned in the anonymized database.

Bear in mind that coded variables possibly underlying an update cannot be used as selection variables when extracting anonymized data for a statistical analysis, because they may have different meanings in different trials due to a change in their coding.

7.5 Security Measures

As mentioned before, the third fundamental step of the anonymization process consists in
- Implementing security measures to prevent a breach of anonymization by simply matching anonymized and respective non anonymized data.

Security of data relates to the "physical" and "logical" protection of personal data by means of organizational and technical measures.

The EU Privacy Directive outlines in its articles 16 and 17 of section VIII the confidentiality and security of processing as follows:

> **SECTION VIII – CONFIDENTIALITY AND SECURITY OF PROCESSING**
> **Article 16 – Confidentiality of processing**
> Any person acting under the authority of the controller or of the processor, including the processor himself, who has access to personal data must not process them except on instructions from the controller, unless he is required to do so by law.
> **Article 17 – Security of processing**
> 1. Member States shall provide that the controller must implement appropriate technical and organizational measures to protect personal data against accidental or unlawful destruction or accidental loss, alteration, unauthorized disclosure or access, in particular where the processing involves the transmission of data over a network, and against all other unlawful forms of processing. Having regard to the state of the art and the cost of their implementation, such measures shall ensure a level of security appropriate to the risks represented by the processing and the nature of the data to be protected.
> 2. The Member States shall provide that the controller must, where processing is carried out on his behalf, choose a processor providing sufficient guarantees in respect of the technical security measures and organizational measures governing the processing to be carried out, and must ensure compliance with those measures.
> 3. The carrying out of processing by way of a processor must be governed by a contract or legal act binding the processor to the controller and stipulating in particular that:
>   - the processor shall act only on instructions from the controller,
>   - the obligations set out in paragraph 1, as defined by the law of the Member State in which the processor is established, shall also be incumbent on the processor.
> 4. For the purposes of keeping proof, the parts of the contract or the legal act relating to data protection and the requirements relating to the measures referred to in paragraph 1 shall be in writing or in another equivalent form.

The measures described above primarily aim at the security of personal data, they do not include special methods necessary to maintain anonymization.

Whenever possible, technical measures should be implemented, but must be supplemented by organizational principles.

Technical measures must take into account the storage of different data types and the subsequent access to different data sources, i.e. the following storage and access principles must be implemented and must be kept under surveillance, i.e. regularly be checked whether the storage and access policies are still met:

Storage Principles

A clear physical separation of data, having different data types, is necessary in order to prevent subjects from uncontrolled merging of clinical and related genetic data, i.e.
- genetic and clinical data must be stored separately from each other.

Recommendation No. R(92) 3 on Genetic Testing and Screening for Health Care Purposes (cf. (15)) defines this requirement as follows:

> **Principle 10 – Separate storage of genetic information**
> Genetic data collected for health care purposes, as for all medical data, should as a general rule be kept separate from other personal records.

(cf. also later, "Storage of Supplementary Information")

In addition, for all data types, i.e. clinical as well as genetic data, a clear physical separation of data having different protection masks must be realized, i.e.
- De-identified and anonymized clinical data must be stored separately from each other.
- De-identified and anonymized genetic data must be stored separately from each other.

Access Principles

Access to data sources having different data types must not be granted.

In addition, for both data types, simultaneous access to data sources having different protection masks must be denied, i.e.
- simultaneous access to anonymized as well as de-identified clinical data must not be granted.
- simultaneous access to anonymized as well as de-identified genetic data must not be granted.

Each subject gets access to one data type at most, i.e. either access to clinical data or access to genetic data, or no access will be granted.

Storage and access principles must be supplemented by organizational measures to provide a complete umbrella of tools to guarantee security of data.

Organizational Principle

It is almost a matter of cause that subjects mostly interested or directly involved in the common evaluation of clinical and related genetic data must not be involved in the specification of security measures for the data they are primarily interested in.

Symbolically speaking: *do not set the fox to watch the geese*

Organizational measures should include but not be limited to:
- Prohibit the matching of anonymized and respective de-identified clinical data by SOPs.
- Prohibit the matching of anonymized and respective de-identified genetic data by SOPs.
- Deny access to both data sources by SOPs, even if a technical solution has already been implemented. SOPs are necessary to close possible technical gaps which are not yet detected.
- Avoid a cumulation of responsibilities, i.e. realize the *distributed responsibilities principle* taking into account *administrative independency*, i.e. subjects responsible for different data types should belong to different administrative units.

Technical measures to be implemented must protect (personal) data against:
- accidental or illegal destruction,
- accidental loss,
- unauthorized access,
- alteration,
- communication or any other form of processing,

and these measures must be reviewed periodically.

The merging of clinical and related genetic data must be implemented as a supervised and controlled process.

We will propose a respective approach in chapter 9 *Request Management*.

As outlined above, the measures discussed so far mainly focus on the physical security of personal data. When handling anonymized data, a new security aspect must be taken into account, i.e. there must be measures in place to guarantee that the anonymized status is maintained.

Everybody involved in the processing of personal data is subjected to the rule of *Data Reduction and Data Economy,* cf. e.g. the Federal Data Protection Act of Germany, Section 3a (cf. (16)). The perfect solution to meet this requirement would be to store personal data only once, and thus avoid data redundancy. However, there may be acceptable reasons to deviate from this basic principle. It is common practice in research to store basic clinical data like age, height, weight, sex, etc together with sample information in laboratory information systems (LIMS). This practice is certainly uncritical as long as anonymization does not play a role in the statistical evaluation strategy. When processsing anonymized data we must take care that there

are no possibilities to breach anonymization, and thus to trace back to the subject's identity. As a rule of thumb:
- the more copies of data exist, the more efforts are necessary to prevent subjects from breaching anonymization by simply matching anonymized data with their de-identified counterparts.

When applying the prespecified/unspecified approach for a clinical study, we start with a prespecified phase, i.e. genetic tests, agreed in the genetic IC, are evaluated as soon as the respective biological material is available and as soon as DNA has been extracted, provided the available genetic IC information is reliable, i.e. genetic IC has been given, genetic IC information has been successfully undergone the source data verification (SDV) process, and the genetic tests specified in the Clinical Trial Protocol (CTP) are admissible, i.e. Ethics Committees involved do not prohibit the conduct of the defined genetic tests.

For further genetic investigations (genetic tests) not yet specified upon start of the study, biological material (e.g. blood, tissue, etc.) or extracted DNA from the same patient must be anonymized and long-term stored in a suitable storage device, e.g. in a special fridge, a biobank or elsewhere. The self-evident question we have to discuss and to answer in this context is:
- How to code aliquots of the same patient, if aliquots are used in both modes, i.e. in prespecified as well as in unspecified mode?

The first convincing approach could be: it is biological material from the same patient, therefore use essentially the same code.

Attaching essentially the same code would mean, however, to relabel each aliquot from the same patient with a unique barcode (nGDI(1), nGDI(2), etc.) and group all these aliquots together via an identical group identifier, a so-called aliquot group number (AGN).

But if we really acted on this advice, the following situation would occur:
- the key relationship **CDI – nGDI(1), AGN** would be stored in the de-identified KPDB for aliquots related to the prespecified phase of the study.
- the key relationship **nCDI – nGDI(2), AGN** would be stored in the anonymized KPDB for aliquots related to the unspecified phase of the study.

Both kinds of aliquots would be related to the same AGN according to the assumption made above, and this would imply that we could trace back to the patient's identity by making use of the CDI – nGDI(1), AGN relationship, stored in the de-identified KPDB, i.e. a breach of anonymization would be possible.

As a first result deduced from these considerations, we can pinpoint:

When collecting samples from one patient for prespecified mode and unspecified mode within the same clinical study, then the AGN codes used in both modes must be different.

But even if we have overcome this first hurdle, may we store supplementary clinical data together with basic sample data? Is this common practice also admissible when processing anonymized data? Well, it is not as simple as it seems to be at the first glance. We will investigate the possible scenarios to get more insight and a better understanding of data handling in an "anonymized environment".

As already mentioned before, it is usually common practice in research to store supplementary clinical information like age, weight, sex, etc. of the patients involved together with basic data of the related samples in a laboratory information system (LIMS). This may be a common procedure as long as the respective LIMS has not been designed for the handling of PGx samples for both modes.

When collecting samples for a de-identified as well as an anonymized phase from the same patient within the same trial, storage of supplementary clinical information with both sample types would lead to a breach of anonymization by simply matching the information related to either sample type. The patient's identity could be revealed without any problems by simply using the nGID(anonymized) – nGDI(de-identified) relationship, and the nGDI(de-identified) – CDI key relationship.

It is therefore necessary to pinpoint:

It is prohibited to store supplementary clinical information with de-identified and anonymized samples simultaneously, to prevent anonymization being broken by simply matching respective record information.

Storing supplementary information with both sample types is counterproductive to anonymization, but has a possible storage of supplementary clinical information with either anonymized or de-identified samples alone the same critical consequences again, namely a breach of anonymization?

When storing supplementary clinical information with anonymized samples only, and provided that de-identified samples of the same patient are also available, the relationship between nCDI and CDI of the same patient could be recognized by relating the de-identified samples to supplementary de-identified information and by simply matching the corresponding de-identified and anonymized information.

It is therefore necessary to pinpoint:

It is prohibited to store supplementary clinical information with anonymized samples.

The last scenario we have to investigate is the possible storage of supplementary clinical information with de-identified samples.

Supplementary clinical information stored with de-identified samples only could be related to the corresponding anonymized information, and the relationship between nCDI and CDI of the same patient could be recognized by matching de-identified and anonymized information.

7 Anonymization

It is therefore necessary to pinpoint:

It is prohibited to store supplementary clinical information with de-identified samples.

In summary:

It is prohibited to store supplementary clinical information with samples.

When working with clinical and genetic data we expect that achieved results of evaluations are without any exception reliable and reproducible. To reach this goal a bundle of measures, required by regulatory authorities and respective laws, must be implemented. We usually speak of validated environments.

A brief introduction to validation is presented in the next section. It is just a reminder for those being familiar with validation, and a first overview for those who never heard of or never applied validation principles before. It is nevertheless a must, a prerequisite for a regulatory submission.

A visualization of the single steps of the anonymization process is given by the diagram in Fig. 7.7.

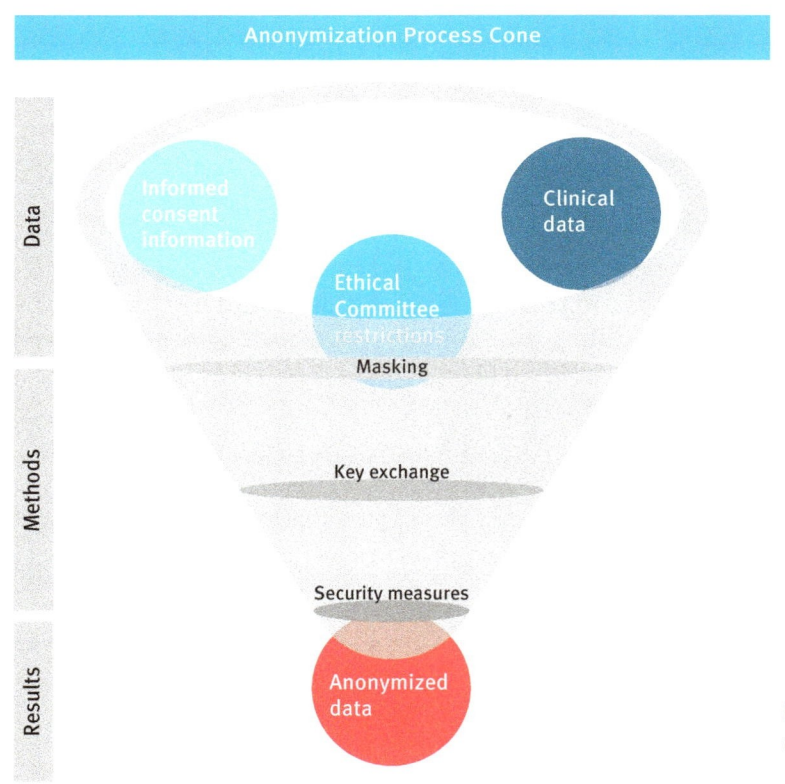

Fig. 7.7 Anonymization Process Cone

8 Validation – a Brief Introduction

8.1 Preliminaries

In the following we describe the basic steps necessary to reach and maintain the validated state of a computerized environment. We will cover only the general principles of the validation process, that is why it is not our intention to provide a complete listing of prescriptive measures in a very narrow sense. We expect that principles provided here are adapted to the special requirements of respective systems to be validated, enhanced or supplemented, if ever adequate.

Numerous guidelines like the *FDA's 21 CFR Part 11, electronic records, electronic signatures*, the *ICH Guideline for Good Clinical Practice E6(R1)* and the *ICH Guideline General Considerations for Clinical Trials E8* illustrate the necessity for validation of computerized systems used in medical environments. We consider validation not only a measure primarily implied by the respective requirements of regulatory authorities, it has moreover been established as a fundamental principle of Good Business Practices. Only permanently controlled, i.e. validated programs and systems provide reliable access to and protection of the most valuable corporate data. Validation is therefore a must beyond doubt.

The attentive reader will easily recognize that data protection and validation have some basic principles in common. Logical and physical access control to systems and thus to data is a matter of course just as the generation of reliable derived data, resulting from different sources. The "equipment" used, i.e. hardware and software components must provide trustworthy, reliable results, and that is only possible if these components did successfully pass a validation process.

8.2 Basic Definitions & Terms

When speaking of computer system validation we must clearly define what is meant by these two notions *computer system* and *validation*.

Computer System
A computer system used in clinical research is defined as:

The set of hardware, software, procedures and people which together perform one or more of the capture, processing, analysis and reporting functions on clinical trials.

(cf. Joint ACDM/PSI Guideline on Computer Systems Validation in Clinical Research, Draft 4 16 September 1997)

Validation

There are numerous definitions of what is meant by validation. Two of them that have regulatory sources are quoted in the following:

> Validation is the process of establishing documented evidence that provides a high degree of assurance that a specific process will consistently produce a product meeting its predetermined specifications and quality attributes.

(cf. FDA, Guidelines on General Principles of Process Validation 1987)
or

> Validation is the collection and evaluation of data, from the process design stage throughout production, which establishes scientific evidence that a process is capable of consistently delivering quality products

(cf. FDA Guidance for Industry – Process Validation: General Principles and Practices, January 2011).
or

> Validation is the demonstration that a computerised system is suitable for its intended purpose.

(cf. OECD, 1995, GLP Consensus Document)

The definition we appreciate most because from our point of view it best meets the real core of what is meant by validation, has been given by Ken Chapman, in 1985

> In today's pharmaceutical industry, whether you are thinking about a computer system, a water treatment system, or a manufacturing process, validation means nothing more than well-organized well-documented common sense.

Unfortunately, sometimes the common sense has been fallen by the wayside.

The main steps of a validation process are often denoted as:
- IQ – **I**nstallation **Q**ualification,
- OQ – **O**perational **Q**ualification,
- PQ – **P**erformance **Q**ualification,

whereby these items are defined as follows:

qualification, installation. (FDA)
Establishing confidence that process equipment and ancillary systems are compliant with appropriate codes and approved design intentions, and that manufacturer's recommendations are suitably considered.

qualification, operational. (FDA)
Establishing confidence that process equipment and sub-systems are capable of consistently operating within established limits and tolerances.

qualification, process performance. (FDA)
Establishing confidence that the process is effective and reproducible.
   (cf. FDA, Glossary of Computer Systems Software Development Terminology, 8/95) http://www.fda.gov/iceci/inspections/inspectionguides/ucm074875.htm

8.3 General Principles of Computer System Validation

Following Ken Chapman's definition of validation we need an organized and structured approach to validation that finalizes each step of the validation process with a detailed documentation of what has to be done, and of what has been done.

The contents and the structure of the validation documents to be compiled can be easily derived by asking and answering the questions:
– What, when, why, who and how?

for each task of the whole validation process.

What is to do?
Describe exactly what is to do, use a step by step approach.

When is it to do?
Describe the context, time points, periods, event triggers, etc. when the distinct tasks must be done.

Why must it be done?
Outline the reasons why a task must be done.

Who actually does it?
Record, who actually performed the respective tasks. Assign responsibilities to distinct tasks. This is absolutely necessary. Bear in mind that

   Tasks do not get done if responsibilities are not assigned to anyone.

How will it be done?
Describe in full detail how the different tasks are to be conducted. For this purpose, provide itemized test plans, checklists, if ever possible and adequate.

All that has been done must be documented in order to provide documented evidence. Store e.g. procedure logs whenever possible and meaningful.

If it ain't documented it ain't done
(Socrates)

Record all responsibilities and let those persons sign the documents to whom responsibility has been assigned for the respective parts of the validation process. These general principles must be applied to all sections of the global validation document.

When to validate? Prior to operational use.

Whether validating prior to the first-time operation of a system or re-validating a computer system, triggered by specific major changes of the validated system, validation should always be executed prior to operational use of the system.
(cf. OECD, 1995, GLP Consensus Document)

How to validate? Pursuant to a formal validation plan.

Validation should be performed by means of a formal validation plan; this reflects a well-organized approach.

Where to validate? Within a test/validation environment.

New releases could disturb running systems, e.g. data may be damaged, if installed changes do not work properly. It is therefore not only a good modus operandi but moreover a must to provide a so-called test environment, where new releases can be primarily installed, tested, and approved. Test/validation and production environment must be essentially the same system, i.e. comparable with respect to hardware, – e.g. hardware from the same vendor, having processors with essentially the same architecture – and as far as possible identical with respect to the system software components involved, ideally a copy of the software environment of the target system.

There is usually no need to physically separate test and production environments. Both may reside on the same hardware but with strictly separated software environments of test and target system, which do not interact with each other.

Independent of the actual status of computer systems waiting for validation, i.e.
- a computer system being already used in production without prior having successfully passed a formal validation procedure, a so-called legacy system,

or
- a computer system not yet released into productive use but still waiting for validation,

the validation process is always conceived as a two-step procedure:
- primary validation – reaching the validated state,

and
- concept for operational use of a computer system – maintaining the validated state.

8.4 Primary Validation – Specification Phase

8.4.1 Introduction

Regulatory authorities require that all computer systems, ranging from single programs to high sophisticated software suites producing data intended to be used in a regulatory submission, must be validated.

The main steps of the whole validation process should always be essentially the same, independent of the different kinds of systems to be validated.

Systems already in use but not yet validated (legacy systems) require a slightly different approach as totally new systems, normally starting from scratch. The validation process for individual programs may be performed by applying agreed programming and validation standards.

All computer systems pass through a SDLC (**S**ystem **D**evelopment **L**ife **C**ycle), including:
- system initiation,
- system development,
- installation,
- productive use, and as a final phase the
- decommissioning, if no longer used.

The validation process on the user's side can be depicted as a three phases model (Fig. 8.1), consisting of:
- A **specification phase** for the system to be developed, including the composition of user requirements, functional requirements, and system design.
- A **preparation phase** of operational use of the new system, i.e. compiling documents, describing the procedures to be implemented for the primary and continuing operational use of the new system.
- A **testing phase** of the new system being provided, including IQ, OQ, and PQ.

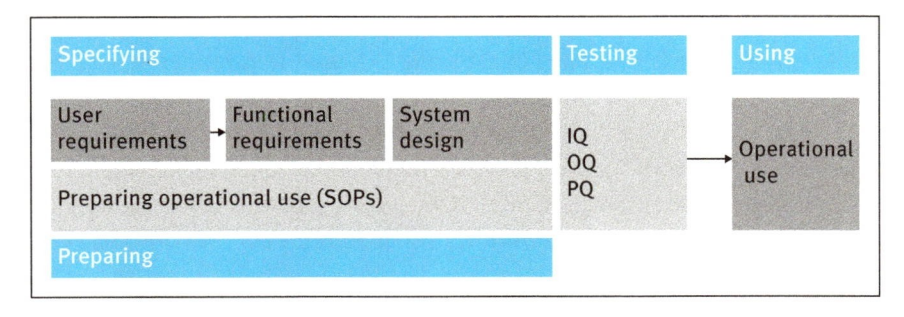

Fig. 8.1 System Development Life Cycle

8.4.2 Preparing User Requirements

Initiation of a new system normally starts with a first rough idea, a basic concept, why and for what purposes a new system should be developed. The intended users are first and foremost responsible for the specification of what they expect from the system to be built and to be implemented. This nontechnical description of the requirements must be provided in a separate document, the user requirements specification. This document should include but not be limited to:
- reasons, why the new system must be installed, e.g. to replace an error-prone manual process, etc.
- a brief description of its intended use, e.g. the main tasks of the new system, the principal users,
- a detailed description of the functionality actually needed, so-called essential requirements,
- a description of desirable requirements, i.e. requirements not necessary for the initial operating of a new system, but nevertheless meaningful, so-called "nice-to have" requirements.

Dependent on the system to be built and the users involved in the specification process, the requirements may vary from a formal description of a program in plain words to the specification of the logical data model, including navigation, access control mechanism, contents and layout of screens and reports as well as logical dependencies between program parts, the definition of logical interfaces to other systems, etc. In any case, it is a nontechnical description from the user's point of view. The essential requirements must be unambiguously defined and testable, because they represent the basis for the User Acceptance Testing, usually referred to as **P**erformance **Q**ualification (**PQ**).

8.4.3 Developing – Functional Requirements

Having successfully finished the phase of defining the user requirements, it is the primary task of the vendor's side to convert the user requirements into functional specifications. This is usually initiated/done by the project leader of the vendor and/ or by an experienced deputy of him. We strongly recommend to do this task in close cooperation with respective representative(s) of the user's side. Our recommendation is based on the experience that without doubt user requirements describe the business processes in question only up to a certain extent, they often do not reveal all internal workflow knowledge necessary to build a new system. What we mean by this is illustrated in the following situation in clinical trials.

Example:
In clinical trials the recruitment of patients usually starts only after the approval of the clinical trial protocol (CTP date), i.e. the date, when the first patient will enter the trial (FPATIN date) is not less than the approval date of the CTP in general. A specification like

"refuse insertion of FPATIN, if FPATIN is less than CTP,"

seems to be correct at the first glance, but would nevertheless be not very meaningful. In phase 1 trials (trials usually initiated by or in the human pharmacological center) recruitment often starts although the clinical trial protocol has not yet been signed. We know from experience that a deferred signing of the CTP may often occur but is due to administrative reasons without exception. A correct translation of this situation into functional specifications is impossible, if this internal knowledge is missing in the user requirements.

It would be better to display a respective message when trying to insert a FPATIN date less than the related CTP date, and let the user decide whether to store the FPATIN date or not. The respective message could be similar to:

*"FPATIN less than CTP, do you still want
to store FPATIN, [yes] or [no]?"*

The user can decide what to do by simply clicking on either button. The system would recognize that *"FPATIN less than CTP"* is an exception, and the involved user would have the possibility to confirm that this exception is nevertheless correct.

Consistency checks of the data must also take into account that those exceptions are likely to occur.

The functional specification should include but not be limited to:
- physical model – data structure, main tables, views, coding tables, definition of ranges, critical values, boundaries, etc.,
- logical program flow charts,
- algorithms, triggers, etc. – only logical definitions, no lines of code are generated at that time,
- screen definitions – naming conventions, layouts, screen navigation,
- concept of access to the system,
- concept of warning and error messages,
- concept for adequate user support – online help on a per screen or per field basis,
- etc.

8.4.4 System Design Specification

The system design specification defines all system components, hardware as well as software, necessary to successfully install and run the new system. In other words, the system design specification must reflect the system topology as a whole. At the latest at installation time a detailed list of suitable environments to successfully run the new system must be available as part of the installation manual, normally provided by the software vendor, including but not limited to,
- central server, network and client hardware, recommended and preferably proved products,
- central server, network and client software, recommended and preferably proved products,
- a step by step procedure to install the application software.

In more detail:
- description of the architecture and configuration of the hardware, including special terminals, local PCs, workstations, specialized printers, e.g. label printers, etc.,
- network components, hardware as well as software,
- peripheral equipment,
- software, databases, querybuilders, interface programs,
- operating systems,
- all components being specifically developed for the new system.

8.4.5 Software Design Specification – System Programming

The definition of the software design specifications as well as the development and primary testing of the individual modules are usually performed by the developer and/or vendor.

The software design specification can be created from the functional requirements, and the system itself can be built from the software design specification.

The user is not directly involved in this process step, but he should ensure that the system is being developed according to commonly accepted standards, in general verified by a vendor audit. This is typically performed by the **Q**uality **A**ssurance (**QA**) of the purchaser (user side).

The software design specification should include but not be limited to:
- description of software development tools, e.g. special open source software,
- programming standards, including guidelines for naming conventions, for code structure, for within code documentation,
- methods, how the source code is maintained, versioning methods, etc.
- source code control mechanism including a plan of which quality checks will be done, when, and how they are to be done.

The contents of all manuals, guidelines to be provided to successfully run the new system must be briefly outlined in addition. This set of documents should include but not be limited to:
- technical manuals,
- user manuals,
- manuals describing the system ergonomics, – GUI, etc.,
- procedure manuals, describing procedures, to be executed by the system, triggers, constraints,
- interface manuals, outlining the communication with other systems.

The complete set of documentation must be available at installation time.

8.5 Primary Validation – Preparing Operational Use

8.5.1 Introduction

Once a computer system has reached the validated state, a substantial set of procedures, rules and measures must be drafted and implemented in order to maintain the validated state. This set of rules and measures is usually referred to as concept for operational use or simply *Operational Concept* and must be in place at the same time when the functional testing, usually denoted as the **O**perational **Q**ualification (**OQ**), is initiated. To reach this goal, all events and factors that might influence the level of validation of the system concerned must be identified and then continuously controlled by means of respective measures.

What may influence the validated state? Well, the definition of a computer system, given at the beginning of the validation section as:

> "... *set of hardware, software, procedures and people ...*"

clearly identifies the main sources that may influence the validated state of a computer system, i.e.:
- hardware,
- software,
- procedures (new or modified, enhanced)
- people.

To maintain the validated state, procedures, covering at least the following areas, must be in place:
- specialized training sessions, to ensure a correct use of the system by different user groups,
- security plan for the system, to protect the system against unauthorized access,

- service and support, to facilitate the daily work with the system, especially upon start,
- monitoring the system, to ensure that the system is operating as supposed,
- error handling, provision of efficient rules and methods to overcome problems in due time,
- backup and restore procedures for application, data, and programs,
- archiving, rules and procedures for long-term storage of data and programs,
- availability management, including disaster and system recovery management, to guarantee the right performance at the right time.

An additional source of variation in the level of validation arises if one or more of these factors are subject to changes. This usually happens if hardware components are replaced or enhanced, system software like operating systems, graphical user interfaces, e.g. Windows-, Unix-or Linux clients, are replaced or upgraded, new database releases are implemented or interface programs to other systems are updated due to a change of other programs communicating with your system. The efficient management of all these changes to a validated system is denoted as **change control**.

All these procedures must be well defined and well documented including assignments of responsibilities to the distinct tasks.

8.5.2 Training

Every user of a system must successfully pass an appropriate preliminary training session prior to getting access to the system for the first time. Appropriate thereby means that the training modules must be stratified according to the different components and tasks of the system, so that potential users can be trained for the correct use of those parts of the system they have been granted access to. Dependent on the respective system, training units for administrators, power users, key users, and normal users should be established at a minimum. Training modules must also be offered if any planned changes in system use occur.

It is recommended to provide the training in entities, as outlined above, headed by qualified personal to ensure users' familiarity with all necessary parts of the system and with any changes made to the system. Training may also be provided or enhanced by e-learning modules. In any case, records of all training activities – who, when, what – of all people involved in the management and/or use of the system must be kept in a separate document.

Manuals in printable and/or electronic form covering all components of the system and all procedures of the application programs must be in place, including but not limited to:
- technical manuals for administrators,

- manuals describing the system ergonomics, e.g. the graphical user interface, drafted for all users,
- application manuals, describing the single tasks, procedures to be applied by the users,
- training manuals.

Releases of respective manuals and subsequent training sessions must be provided as soon as changes to the system application have been made, but prior to operational use of those changes.

In addition, all items used, i.e. procedures, policies, and all kind of manuals must be complete and current.

8.5.3 Security Management

It is a matter of course that only authorized users should have access to hardware, software and/or data of a computer system. The system itself must be protected against corruption and accidental loss of data. The implementation and application of the complete bundle of measures and procedures enabling the realization of these requirements is usually referred to as security management. It is without any doubt a necessary must in order to keep the integrity of the system and to furthermore guarantee its validated state.

Two different aspects of security must be covered by the implemented security management:
- the logical security,

and
- the physical security

of the system, whereby logical security methods are rules and measures managing the prevention of unauthorized access to respective systems, software, and application programs.

Measures and procedures to be established should cover but not be limited to the following areas:
- Rules and responsibilities for assigning access rights to all components of the system, hardware – servers, clients, network – system software and application. It is important to know who has when what level of access to which parts of the system.

  The grantors of rights as well as the grantees must be documented, stratified according to the system components mentioned above, and user profiles assigned like administrators, key users, superusers, normal users etc. Keeping track of access rights is possible if and only if access rights are granted without grant options, i.e. the single user must not be enabled to grant his own access rights to other subjects without the explicit agreement of the system owner.

- Regular review of access rights and responsibilities to ensure that they are still appropriate.
- Rules for password definition and methods for regular change.
- System protection from all kinds of viruses.
- Implementation of intruder detection methods.
- Security of electronic links to transfer data, generally including firewalls, VPNs (**V**alue **P**rivate **N**etworks), SSL (**S**ecure **S**ockets **L**ayer), TSL (**T**ransport **L**ayer **S**ecurity), FTP (**F**ile **T**ransfer **P**rotocol), sFTP (**s**ecure **F**ile **T**ransfer **P**rotocol), AES (**A**dvanced **E**ncryption **St**andard) encryption algorithm, etc., if adequate.

Rules and measures established to prevent subjects from non-authorized physical access to the computer system hardware are referred to as physical security procedures. These procedures should include but not be limited to:
- protection of clients, e.g. screen savers, automatically invoked after a certain time of non-processing, lockable devices, etc.,
- access control mechanism to facilities, e.g. card access to computer rooms, biometric identification, etc.,
- special sign in procedures.

In addition, an itemized documentation must be in place that tracks who has which kind of access to which components of the system during which time period.

Supplementary measures must be established, dependent on the intended use of the installed system, e.g. a separate and lockable room is required when using a clinical labeling system.

8.5.4 Service and Support

A concept in which way and to what extent service and support will be provided to the users and staff should be available, covering but not limited to the following areas:
- key user concept, if applicable,
- provision of manuals (as printout or electronically),
- online help system, on a per screen and/or on per field basis,
- help desk, including support strategy for remote users, if adequate,
- vendor hotline established for key users and administrators.

8.5.5 Monitoring

To guarantee the accessibility of a computer system and the reliability of obtained results, all critical components of the system like hardware, software, and application programs must be identified and monitored regularly. Hardware failures in general appear gradually, apart from some extreme critical events like head crashes, software failures however usually occur unexpectedly without advanced warning. A systematic monitoring of the system and of all critical system processes enables a premature detection of failures and incidents, so that prospective measures for replacing respective components can be initiated prior to a necessary shut down of the application. Measures to be in place should cover all components of the system, whereby a regular check of all system and application logfiles is a must. Supplementary and enhanced monitoring methods like process and performance monitoring should be offered and should be available on request.

8.5.6 Error Handling – Problem Management

Procedures to manage and in particular to solve all known and new problems arising during installation, updating, upgrading or operational use of a computer system must be implemented. At a minimum these procedures must cover methods for:
- Reporting of problems – who reports to whom, in which way, and when?
- Recording of reported problems – establishing a problem or bug database with controlled access.
- Resolution of problems – agreed timeframes for availability of workarounds, patches, updates and/or upgrades.

8.5.7 Backup and Restore Management

Backup and restore procedures for software and data must have been implemented to guarantee that a valid and reliable state of the system can be provided at any time. The procedures to be implemented must cover but not be limited to:
- Description of the backup procedure, including hardware, e.g. dedicated hard discs, SAN (**S**torage **A**rea **N**etwork), software, e.g. backup software, allowing the storage of backup related keywords to easier select data for a necessary retrieval, and procedural approach, e.g. online – offline backup.
- The documentation of all backup requests, i.e. who initiated, what, and when.
- The itemized documentation of all backup activities, including the check and, if adequate, storage of backup logs, error reports, etc..
- Detailed backup plans for periodical, full, and incremental backups.
- Agreements with the potential users of the system upon reasonable times for restoration of distinct parts of the system.

8.5.8 Archiving

Data not been accessed during a well-defined time period should be removed from the running system, not simply deleted but rather long-term stored, to provide an optimal and enhanced system performance. This process is usually referred to as archiving. Methods and/or tools designed for archiving should cover at least but not be limited to the following areas:
- Long-term storage of data and programs.
- Fast and reliable retrieval on demand. Prerequisite is the classification of objects to be archived by keywords in a respective database.
- Data conversion to new system standards in the context of application changes and decommissioning.

In addition, there must be rules in place with respect to when, and what to archive, e.g. archiving the current system prior to implementing new releases, patches, etc.

8.5.9 Availability Management

Prior to productive use of a system there should be an agreement in place upon the necessary and required availability of the system, covering but not limited to the following areas:
- Time frames, when the system is available without any restrictions.
- Guaranteed system performance, e.g. average and greatest expected response time in the context of database requests.
- System layout, including redundancy of critical components, e.g. disk mirroring, several I/O channels, etc..
- Disaster management. What happens when the system crashes? Are there approved procedures in place to recover the system in due time?
- The possibility of switching to 'backup systems', i.e. alternative site(s), if meaningful and appropriate.

In addition, preventive methods to handle emergency situations like:
- fire,
- earthquake,
- sabotage,
- power supply breakdown,
- etc.,

should be in place, if adequate.

8.5.10 Change Control Management

During its lifecycle each system is subject to changes that may or may not influence the validated state. It is therefore necessary to establish procedures in order to manage changes to be made to the computer system. Those changes may occur with respect to:
- Hardware configurations, – complete or partial replacement of equipment and/or components.
- Software configuration, – new releases, updates, upgrades, patches.
- People, staff and/or users, and
- procedures (application software).

All executed changes must be documented, and respective records must "answer" the question *"who, what, why, when and how"* for each change made to the system, i.e.:
- Who did authorize the changes?
- What has been changed?
- Why have changes been made?
- When have the changes been done?
- How have changes been done, tested and released into production?

In addition, a version control of all component changes made must be in place, in order to be able to unambiguously track which configuration was implemented during which time period. Regulatory authorities often ask for the software environment, application names and releases which have been used at evaluation time. Management and documentation of changes of the system configuration are often referred to as configuration management.

New or enhanced does not necessarily mean better or improved. The appropriateness of the modified environment must always be proved. The impact on the validated state of each change made to the system must be evaluated.

What kind of changes trigger which level of re-testing (re-evaluation) or re-validation of what part of the system? To ensure that the system will continue to do what it is expected to do, respective measures must be initiated and performed covering but not limited to:
- Testing of changes.
- Interactions with other parts of the system.
- Complementary training for all people involved.

8.5.11 Periodic Review of Computer Systems

Systems that are not subject to systematic and/or planned changes may yet have a varying state of validation. There are always unknown influences on the system components that can never be entirely controlled by systematic procedures.

A risk analysis to point out all critical points of the system should be performed and a re-evaluation of those critical points having a decreasing reliability must be initiated after reasonable time.

8.5.12 Decommissioning of Computer Systems

Procedures must be in place that manage the decommissioning of systems. The most important task in this phase of the SDLC is to provide strategies for subsequent access to archived data. Software and hardware technologies are subject to substantial changes within short time periods, that is why methods for data and software storage independent of individual, proprietary hardware architectures and file structures are to be preferred. A loss of data may occur, if stored and archived data are not converted to the appropriate format standard.

8.6 Primary Validation – Testing Phase

8.6.1 Installation Qualification

Each new system release and all changes intended to be made to a production system must at first be installed and tested within a test environment. Test and production environment must be in compliance with the environments the software has been designed for.

The documented evidence that the equipment and system as installed or modified are in conformity with the approved design and the recommendations of the vendor is denoted as **Installation Qualification** (**IQ**). This is the first step of the validation process.

The actual installation plan, provided by the personnel which actually does the installation, should include but not be limited to:
- A diagram, flowchart of the network topology, covering the distinct components of the system, the system configuration plan.
- Hardware installation plan.
- Installation plan of system software, e.g. operating systems, network and interface software.
- Software installation plan, describing how the system has been installed, including a listing of default settings at installation time.

- A complete and signed checklist, revealing that the whole installation procedure is in accordance with the specifications.

In addition, the following tasks must have been done:
- A check that all technical manuals, needed for primary installation, customization, operating and administration of the system are in place and have been updated to the latest standard.
- A check that the complete documentation for the potential users of the system has been provided.
- A check that the helpdesk for the new system has been initiated, if appropriate.
- A check whether administrator and potential key users of the new system have successfully passed a preliminary training.
- A check whether training modules for different user profiles have been provided, e.g. special training sessions for advanced users, planned to get access to a querybuilder.

8.6.2 Operational Qualification – Functional Testing

Operational **Q**ualification (**OQ**) is the verification that the system meets all characteristics as defined in the functional requirements. The goal of the OQ therefore is the confirmation that all functions, necessary for the intended use, have been provided and operate reliably in the target environment. It is recommended that this qualification at the user's site will be conducted by the vendor and/or user in close cooperation, if possible. Preferably automated OQ test scripts prepared by the vendor will be executed by the vendor/user at the user's site. Test results are reviewed, documented and signed. The single steps of an OQ should cover the following areas:
- Development of a test plan that encompasses the functionality of the system as required by the functional requirements.
- Development of test cases for all items described in the functional requirements, documented in the functional test manual. Test cases should be reviewed by the user to ensure that sufficient testing is taken into account.
- Executing the tests and documenting the achieved results on the respective sheets of the functional test manual.
- Summarizing the results in the functional test report manual.

In more detail, for each item, procedure, described in the functional requirements, tests must be developed in order to check the desired and agreed functionality of the system.

The test cases should cover all critical points and parameters of the system to be tested, and all special
- features not to be tested,
- features to be tested,

including limits for critical points to be tested as well as valid and invalid test cases. For each test case the following uniform test structure is recommended:
- Description of what will be tested.
- Description in which way it will be tested, i.e. test approach, test instruction, including item "pass/fail" – criteria.
- Input data, if applicable.
- Expected output data, if applicable.

To check how the system handles correct and incorrect input, the test data should include:
- representative data, realistic file sizes, etc.,
- extreme values,
- boundary values,
- missing values,
- incorrect values, e.g. specify a wrong password for password protected modules, monitor and document how the system reacts.

After having tested, the test sheets should be completed with:
- The actual output, if applicable.
- The test results according to the item "pass/fail" – criteria. Recommended categories are e.g. "pass", "conditional pass" and "failure".
- Comments with respect to the test results, recording anomalies and possible resolutions, if applicable.
- Date and time when the test has been executed.
- Signature(s) of the tester(s).
- Date and time when tests have been reviewed, if applicable.
- Signature(s) of the reviewer(s), if applicable.

An overall summary of the functional tests with a conclusion as to acceptability of the results should be provided as a separate document, the functional test report.

Validation from its very nature is in the first instance a prospective measure. Nevertheless, there are many systems already used in production without prior having passed a formal validation procedure, so-called legacy systems. To attain the validated state for a legacy system, all methods normally applied to prospective validation processes must also be applied to legacy systems with necessary adaptations; i.e. all steps to reach the validated state must be executed retrospectively.

8.6.3 Performance Qualification – User Acceptance Testing

Performance **Q**ualification (**PQ**) is the confirmation that a system meets the specified requirements and works reliably in a production environment.

To prove the required functionality a test procedure similar to that of an Operational Qualification must be defined and executed. Test cases are derived from the user requirements, and the single test steps are exclusively performed by the user. The vendor is not primarily involved in the Performance Qualification. It is recommended to delegate the Performance Qualification to several power users, in order to be able to guarantee with a clear conscience that all aspects of the system have been sufficiently tested. Performance Qualification is usually referred to as User Acceptance Testing.

The procedural methods to be applied are similar to those applied during an Operational Qualification. Test plan and test cases must be developed and documented in an user acceptance test manual. Tests must be conducted, documented, signed and the complete test results must be summarized in an user acceptance test report (Fig. 8.2).

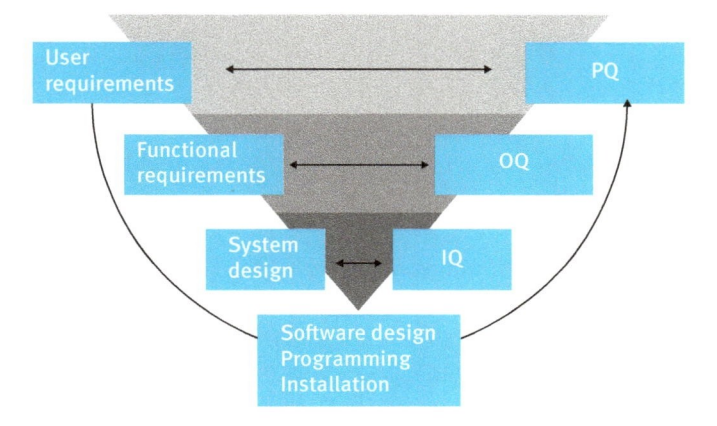

Fig. 8.2 System Development & Validation

8.6.4 Off the Shelf Systems

Commercial systems, standard software packages usually provide more features and more procedures than actually needed and actually used. A complete validation of those systems would make no sense, it would be a waste of validation efforts.

It is therefore a good strategy, implied by the correct understanding of validation, to validate the computer system only to a certain extent, to specific processes, or expressed in the language of validation, only for its intended use. The expected functionality of the system to be installed must be described in full detail.

Specify what you want, what you need, and what you are expecting from the system. Use the following approach:
- Identify the processes actually needed and intended to be used.
- Outline and document those processes, nothing less but also nothing more.

- Validate the system only up to the required functionality.
- Restrict the use of the system to the validated part, either by technical measures, if applicable, and/or by respective SOPs.

8.6.5 Risk Analysis

An error free system is almost impossible to attain; there is always a remaining risk that deviations from a required functionality occur, varying from a partial up to a complete breakdown. You should be aware of the possible consequences of breakdowns, i.e. you should develop a knowledge about the impact of such breakdowns on your business processes, or in other words, you should be able to estimate the risk with respect to your business processes if a special feature fails.

A first but already good impression of possible risk scenarios can be gained by performing a formal risk analysis. Expected failures are judged according to the two characteristics *frequency or likelihood of occurrence*, and *severity level*, i.e.:
- how often do we expect a system feature to fail, and
- what is the severity level of a system feature failure with respect to the business processes?

The likelihood that a special component will not work is often difficult to estimate. A good and usually sufficient stratification is given by use of a three point ordinal scale with classes *"low"*, *"medium"*, and *"high"*. The severity level of the impact of a failure on business processes is essentially easier to estimate; the possible consequences are often already known or can be determined in due time. We recommend a four point ordinal scale with classes *"no"*, *"low"*, *"medium"*, and *"high"*. Likelihood of occurrence and severity of failure are visualized in a 3 x 4 contingency table (Fig. 8.3):

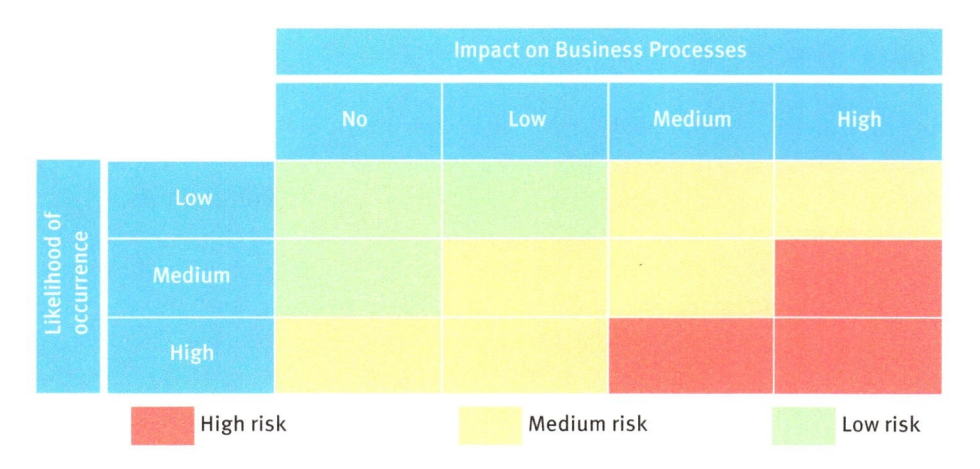

	Impact on Business Processes			
Likelihood of occurrence	No	Low	Medium	High
Low	Low risk	Low risk	Medium risk	Medium risk
Medium	Low risk	Medium risk	Medium risk	High risk
High	Medium risk	Medium risk	High risk	High risk

Fig. 8.3 Business Risk Table

Business risk is a function of severity (impact on business processes), and frequency (likelihood of occurrence), i.e.
   risk = f(severity, frequency),
while the mapping of "(severity, frequency)" pairs to risk classes is highly dependent on the special business situation under consideration. An example for a possible mapping is given above.

Events with high business impact but low probability of occurrence that gradually appear may have a lower risk assessment than events having a medium impact on business, a high probability of occurrence but an abrupt appearance, i.e. the time up to the appearance of an event, the lead time, is an important factor for the final risk assessment.
– The longer the time to react, the lower the actual risk, and this implies:
– risk = f(severity, frequency, lead time)

This comprehension of risk management implies that it is absolutely necessary,
– to discover all sources of risk prematurely,
– to assess the risk level,
– to permanently survey potential sources of risk,
– to define measures to be executed, if potential risk has been detected prior to breakdown of the system.

The steps outlined above should be performed for the user as well as for the functional requirements, documented, signed, and compiled in respective risk assessment manuals.

8.6.6 Traceability of Results

A fundamental requirement all validation processes must meet, is the traceability of obtained results, i.e. the relationships between user requirements, acceptance test cases, and the related risk assessments must be documented as well as the relationships between functional requirements, functional test cases, and the respective risk assessments. It may happen that some requirements are related to several test cases, e.g. the user requirement "*the system must be able to handle incorrect values*" usually implies more than one test case, dependent on the kind of incorrect values specified. How this *one to many relationship* between user requirements and user requirements test cases can be numbered consecutively, is demonstrated in Fig. 8.4.

Traceability Table : URs – UR Test Cases – Risk Analysis		
User requirement no.	UR test case no.	Risk analysis no.
UR0001	URT0001	URA0001
UR0002	URT0002	URA0002
UR0003	URT0003_1	URA0003_1
	URT0003_2	URA0003_2
⋮		
UR0020	URT0020	URA0020
⋮		

Fig. 8.4 Traceability Table URs – UR Test Cases – Risk Analysis

Between user requirements test cases and the related risk assessments exists always a *one to one relationship.*

The relationships between functional requirements, functional test cases and the respective risk assessments can be handled in essentially the same way. A suitable numbering schema is given in Fig. 8.5.

Traceability Table : FRs – FR Test Cases – Risk Analysis		
Functional requirement no.	FR test case no.	Risk analysis no.
FR0001	FRT0001	FRA0001
FR0002	FRT0002	FRA0002
FR0003	FRT0003_1	FRA0003_1
	FRT0003_2	FRA0003_2
⋮		
FR0020	FRT0020	FRA0020
⋮		

Fig. 8.5 Traceability Table FR – FR Test Cases – Risk Analysis

The proposed schema is self-explanatory so that a separate documentation is not really necessary from our point of view (Fig. 8.6).

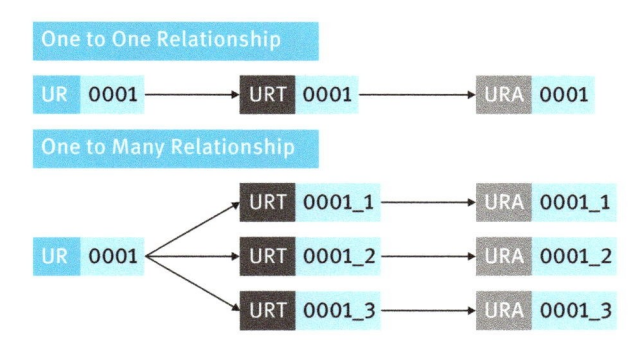

Fig. 8.6 Numbering Schema

Our recommendation:

> *Keep it simple, it's not a scientific discipline, but rather well-organized, well-documented common sense.*

8.6.7 Validation Report

The final step of the validation process, conducted so far, consists in the compilation of a validation report, providing an overall judgment of all results obtained. Any deviation occurred must be discussed, respective conclusions must be drawn, and measures to correct observed deficiencies must be established.

9 Request Management

The anonymization process has been designed as the three entities approach, briefly referred to as the **SDK** (**S**ample, **D**ata, **K**ey) approach, and this modus operandi induces in a natural way how a common analysis of anonymized clinical and related genetic data must be initiated, i.e. the necessary merging of both data sources can only, namely exclusively, be performed on request by the **K**ey **P**rotection **D**ata**B**ase. Users interested in such a genetic analysis must file a formal request, which must be checked for admissibility and meaningfulness by an independent internal committee. Details why and how such a committee must be established will be explained below.

9.1 Genetic Review Board (GRB)

When applying prespecified mode, all genetic tests to be carried out must be specified in advance, i.e. prior to the start of the clinical trial, and the intended tests can be only performed if and only if they have been released by the competent Ethics Committees.

The situation in evaluating anonymized clinical and related genetic data is slightly different, because the planning of statistical evaluations can be initiated only after closure of a trial, i.e. patients to be included in such an analysis are often related to trials, not necessarily only one, which are already finished and reported.

Ethics Committees can, and often do so, impose restrictions on future genetic analyses involving anonymized samples, these might be e.g. restrictions to the therapeutic area the test drug is related to or even restrictions to the indication, but in general there is no further impact of Ethics Committees on "anonymized" evaluations planned with anonymized clinical and related genetic data. A survey of those kinds of analyses is rather an internal than an external process. It is therefore recommendable to establish an internal and independent committee as the anonymized counterpart of the external Ethics Committee.

This independent committee should decide upon the meaningfulness and admissibility of an intended common analysis of anonymized clinical and related genetic data. This committee will be referred to as

Genetic **R**eview **B**oard (**GRB**) in the following.

The primary tasks of the GRB can be briefly summarized as:
- Responsibility for checking and releasing or denying a request for a common statistical evaluation of anonymized clinical and related genetic data, i.e. the GRB must review provided requests with respect to concept and admissibility, and with respect to scientific, and technical issues, taking into account medical, genetic, statistical, and data protection aspects. The proof of feasibility of the request with respect to strategic and financial aspects does not belong to the primary responsibilities of the GRB.

The constitution of the GRB members should be well-balanced with respect to the different disciplines involved in the genetic area, i.e. GRB should include at least
- one representative of Medicine,
- one representative of Genetics, mostly from Research & Development,
- one representative of Data Protection/Medicine, familiar with statistical methods, and
- one biostatistician, having at least a good knowledge of genetics and statistical methods to be suitable in this area.

9.2 Request Specification

Information to be provided by a requester to the Key Protection DataBase must include but not be limited to:

Scientific Issues
- An itemized and comprehensible description of the intended common statistical evaluation of anonymized clinical and related genetic data.
- The specification of a so-called *"patient pattern"*, describing characteristics of patients whose clinical data (clinical records) are to be included in the statistical evaluation. Based on this information the number of patients with samples available for genetic testing purposes can be determined.
- The listing of attributes (variables) to be included.

Alternatively, this can be also included in the statistical analysis plan as a separate section.
- A statistical analysis plan, outlining the statistical analysis to be applied, including a sample size estimation for the intended analysis. Remember that a statistical analysis plan for these purposes is not yet available, as we plan an "anonymized" evaluation.
- A specification of genetic tests including necessary result formats, to be applied to the samples selected.
- A specification of the therapeutic area and indication, if adequate, which the genetic tests to be carried out are related to. This information is needed in order to check for Ethics Committee restrictions and in order to meet them.
- Number of matched ICs compared to therapeutic area and indication.

Financial Issues
- An estimation of expected costs for the genetic tests to be carried out; taking into account whether internal or external laboratories must be involved.

- Specification of the time frame and timelines, when intended analysis should be done. This is necessary for resources planning – internal labs versus external labs, statistical evaluation, internally or externally.

This information must be provided by a requester but is by no means sufficient in order to decide upon the adequacy of a request. The GRB needs some more information prior to coming to a final decision. Supplementary information to a request must be prepared by the Key Protection DataBase and will be sent together with the original request to the GRB.

The supplementary information to be provided is essentially a list of clinical studies involved, containing:
- the respective study numbers,
- the number of patients per study, and
- the number of patients selected, i.e. the number of all patients having samples that may be included in the planned genetic analysis.

The GRB must take into account sizes of selected studies, and especially the number of selected patients for genetic analysis on a per study and a per center in study basis to guarantee that a breach of anonymization is not possible due to too small population sizes.

Example of patient pattern
"All female patients older than 20, being non-smoker, and having a weight over 100 kg should be included in a genetic analysis."

Criterion 1: female patients, used variable: *sex*
Criterion 2: patients with an age > 20 used variable: *age*
Criterion 3: non-smoker, used variable: *smoking behavior*
Criterion 4: weight over 100 kg, used variable: *weight*.

Another patient pattern would be:
"All patients from Study 123"

Criterion 1: study_number="123" used variable: *study_number*

In case that a request has been accepted, several further steps must be initiated.
- The list of selected sample identifiers nGDI together with the list of genetic tests to be performed must be sent to the responsible institution, in general the respective laboratory information system for PGX samples, for further processing, i.e. DNA samples must be selected from the storage device, and specified genetic tests must be performed.

We strongly recommend a check prior to the performance of any genetic test as to whether specified genetic tests have already been conducted with other requests and whether respective results for at least some of the selected samples (nGDIs) are thus already available and usable. Such a prior check for genetic results must be performed by the institution where genetic test results are stored, i.e. by the anonymized genetic data base.
- A check for existence of genetic test results will save time and resources.

The genetic test results related to a request are securely stored in the anonymized genetic database and also sent to the Key Protection DataBase for further processing.
The next step to be done by the KPDB is
- to retrieve the anonymized clinical data related to the current request.

Remember that the KPDB exclusively stores the key relationship between anonymized clinical data and related samples/genetic data. It now owns the request related anonymized clinical data, the request related genetic data, and the key relationship between them, i.e. the nCDI – nGDI relationship.

When specifying the single steps of the anonymization process, we emphasized that merging of both data sources can only, namely exclusively, be performed on request by the Key Protection DataBase. This implies that the key relationship nCDI – nGDI will never leave the Key Protection DataBase KPDB. This however means that available anonymized clinical and related genetic data must be slightly modified with respect to their identifiers to retain the original key information nCDI – nGDI exclusively in the KPDB.

It is the task of the KPDB:
- to exchange the nCDI identifier of the anonymized clinical data with a new **r**equest **C**linical **D**ata **I**dentifier **rCDI**,
- to exchange the nGDI identifier of the anonymized genetic data with a new **r**equest **G**enetic **D**ata **I**dentifier **rGDI**, and
- to replace the original key relationship nCDI – nGDI by the new key relationship **rCDI – rGDI**.

The new identifiers rCDI and rGDI are strictly request related, i.e. if the same sample is selected by distinct requests, then the respective identifiers are also different. This implies:
- The key relationship between anonymized clinical data and related genetic data provided on a per request basis does not reveal the original key relationship of anonymized clinical data and related samples/genetic data, exclusively held by the KPDB.

Merging of anonymized clinical and related genetic data cannot be done without the support of the KPDB, and this support will only be granted on the basis of an available request, released by the Genetic Review Board.

Having successfully passed the key exchange process nCDI → rCDI, and nGDI → rGDI, anonymized clinical as well as related genetic data, and the rCDI − rGDI key relationship can now be provided to a **S**ecure **E**valuation **A**rea (**SEA**) for evaluation purposes.

How a SEA must be set up depends primarily on the software environment used. In any case, there must be security measures in place that prevent a breach of anonymization by simply matching anonymized data with their de-identified counterparts. In addition, it is recommended that data subjects mainly working with de-identified clinical data must not be involved in the evaluation of anonymized data.

In summary:

An itemized request management stores the complete audit trail information of:
- Who required which kind of genetic analysis, and when.
- Who released what, and when.
- Who triggered what, and when.
- What has been done, and
- when was it done.

9.3 Subrequest Specification

The results of a common statistical evaluation of anonymized clinical and related genetic data often trigger new questions that should be answered in addition, i.e. there may be supplementary genetic tests necessary to be carried out with a subpopulation of the population selected so far with the request, whereas the anonymized clinical data selected with the original request remain unchanged.

How should we proceed in this special case?

Well, apply essentially the same procedure, i.e. provide a subrequest to the KPDB containing basically the same elements as already specified in the original request. Omit elements like the specification of the therapeutic area that will not change within a subrequest.

The GRB must be involved again. It has to decide whether the submitted subrequest is admissible, taking into account that additional genetic tests are now requested to be carried out with a smaller population (Fig. 9.1).

Supplementary genetic data generated with a subrequest are stored in the anonymized genetic database and also sent to the KPDB for further processing.

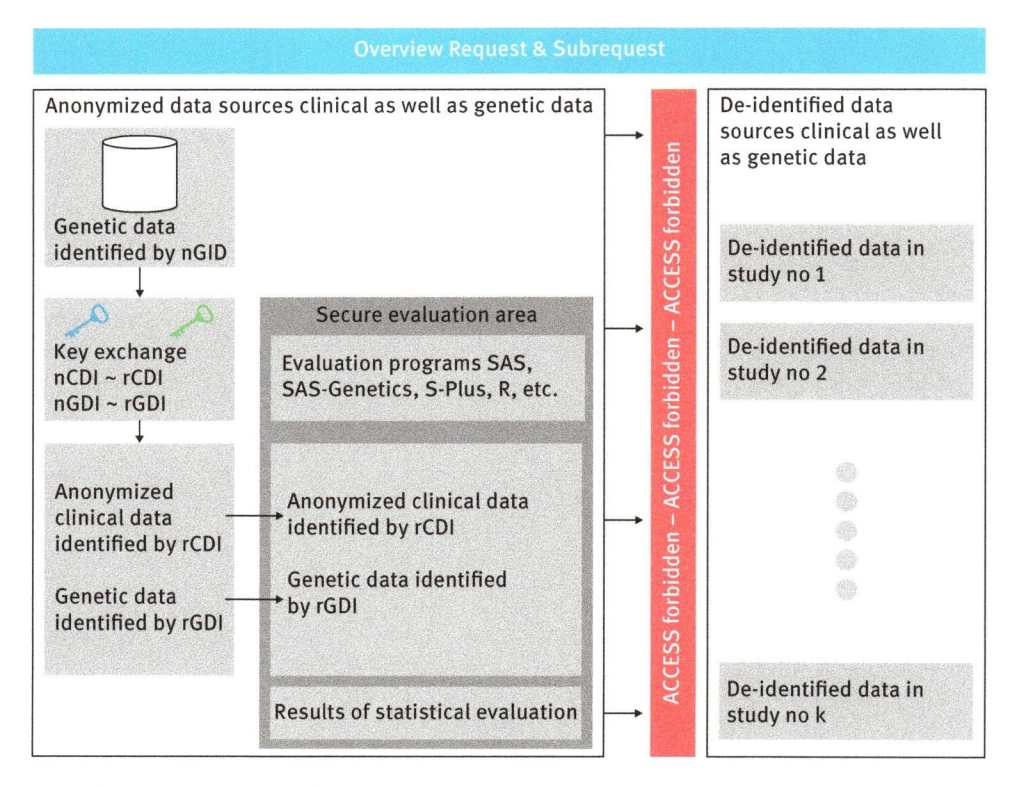

Fig. 9.1 Overview Request and Subrequest

The KPDB replaces the nGDI identifier of the genetic data with the respective rGDI identifier already generated with the original request, i.e. the request genetic data identifier of any subrequest of a request is identical to the respective rGDI of the original request.

Remember: we do not add new samples within a subrequest but perform only new genetic tests with already selected samples.

9.4 Involvement of External Service Providers

Involving external service providers in the DNA extraction process or in the evaluation of genetic tests would reveal internal coding standards to contracted research organizations (CROs). The primary linking code of samples to the respective data is the nGDI barcode, attached to the blood samples upon sample registration at the sponsor's site.

Blood samples labeled with a nGDI barcode are delivered to a CRO for DNA extraction. Those involved CROs must agree that storage of the nGDI code on their local devices is prohibited (Fig. 9.2).

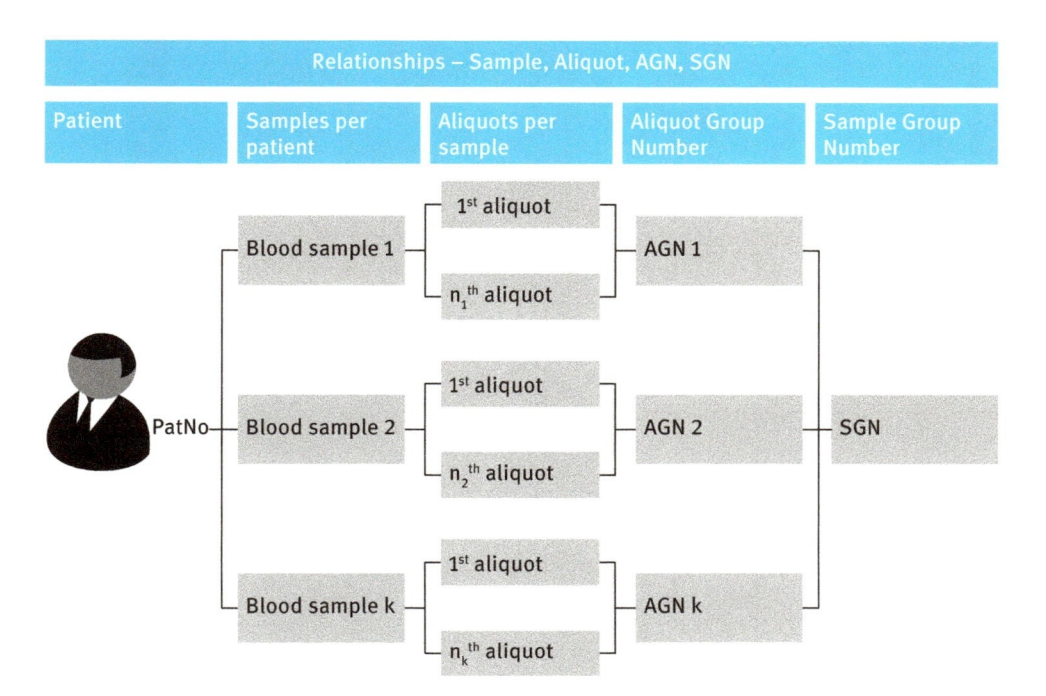

Fig. 9.2 Relationships between Samples, Aliquots, AGN and SGN

In addition, we must guarantee that the primary sample code, internally used, never leaves the sponsor company. This can be reached by exchanging the original nGDI code for a newly generated unique random code upon receipt of the extracted DNA and the accompanying quality data.

Remember that DNA samples delivered by a service provider are no longer directly identified by the original nGDI. The individual samples (aliquots) are usually identified by a different barcode, e.g. a 2D barcode, dependent on the DNA storage device used. The new code relationships between original nGDI and related DNA aliquots is provided by the external extraction laboratory (CRO), stored in the Key Protection DataBase (KPDB) upon receipt, and subsequently the original nGDI is replaced by a new one.

Applying this procedure guarantees that the **K**ey **P**rotection **D**ata**B**ase is the only instance that knows the relationship between the original blood samples and the related DNA samples.

DNA samples extracted by a contracted external service provider are created prior to the start of the anonymization process. All data associated with the DNA aliquots are still personal data and are therefore subjected to the respective data protection legislative. In Germany, the extraction process described would be governed by section 11 "*Collection, processing or use of personal data on behalf of others*" of the Federal Data Protection Act (BDSG) as of 1 September 2009 with amendments 2010. The controller, i.e. the representative of the customer (sponsor) is subjected to comprehensive data protection obligations. He is responsible for the compliance with the provisions of the BDSG. Sponsor and service provider should be aware of the scope and importance of section 11 of the BDSG.

Section 11 Collection, processing or use of personal data on behalf of others
(1) If other bodies collect, process or use personal data on behalf of the controller, the controller shall be responsible for compliance with the provisions of this Act and other data protection provisions. The rights referred to in Sections 6, 7 and 8 shall be asserted with regard to the controller.
(2) The processor shall be chosen carefully, with special attention to the suitability of the technical and organizational measures applied by the processor. The work to be carried out by the processor shall be specified in writing, including in particular the following:
   1. the subject and duration of the work to be carried out,
   2. the extent, type and purpose of the intended collection, processing or use of data, the type of data and category of data subjects,
   3. the technical and organizational measures to be taken under Section 9,
   4. the rectification, erasure and blocking of data,
   5. the processor's obligations under subsection 4, in particular monitoring,
   6. any right to issue subcontracts,
   7. the controller's rights to monitor and the processor's corresponding obligations to accept and cooperate,
   8. violations by the processor or its employees of provisions to protect personal data or of the terms specified by the controller which are subject to the obligation to notify,
   9. the extent of the controller's authority to issue instructions to the processor,
   10. the return of data storage media and the erasure of data recorded by the processor after the work has been carried out.

In case of public bodies, the work to be carried out may also be specified by the authority responsible for expert supervision. The controller shall verify compliance with the technical and organizational measures taken by the processor before data processing begins and regularly thereafter. The result shall be documented.

(3) The processor may collect, process or use the data only as instructed by the controller. If the processor believes that an instruction by the controller violates this Act or other data protection provisions, the processor shall inform the controller of this immediately.
(4) For the processor, other than Sections 5, 9, 43 (1) no. 2, Sections 10 and 11 (2) nos. 1 through 3 and (3), and Section 44, only the provisions on data protection monitoring or supervision shall apply, namely for
   1. a) public bodies,
      b) private bodies, when the majority of shares or votes is publicly owned and the controller is a public body, Sections 18, 24 through 26 or the corresponding provisions of the data protection laws of the Länder,
   2. other private bodies, where they collect, process or use personal data on behalf of others for commercial purposes as service providers, Sections 4f, 4g and 38.
(5) Subsections 1 through 4 shall apply accordingly if other bodies carry out the inspection or maintenance of automated procedures or data processing systems and the possibility of access to personal data during such inspection and maintenance cannot be ruled out.

For detailed information cf. (17). Cf. also chapter 13 *"Impact of External Services on Data Protection"*.

10 Legal Requirements & Regulations

10.1 Basic Ideas

When conducting clinical trials involving human subjects we implicitly adopt the principles outlined in the Nuremberg Code of 1947 (cf. App 4), the World Medical Association's Declaration of Helsinki of 1964, and the subsequent revisions of it. In addition, we are subjected to a multitude of legal requirements and regulations that must be met without any exception. For example, Good Clinical Practice is strictly regulated by the European DIRECTIVE 2001/20/EC of 4 April 2001 (cf. (18)).

During the conduct of clinical trials numerous sensitive personal data of the human subjects involved will be created that require a particularly careful handling, usually realized by implementing and periodically monitoring adequate data protection and data security measures. Principles to be applied in this context are by no means left to the discretion of the responsible study sponsor, but are rather regulated by international and local laws, almost without exception but dependent on and varying with the countries where the respective trials are conducted.

The central pillar of data protection in the European Union is the EU Privacy Directive obliging all EU member states to implement national data protection laws providing at least the same data protection standards or even data protection standards going beyond. Dependent on the federal structure of some member states also regional data protection laws of respective countries must be taken into account when processing personal data (Fig. 10.1).

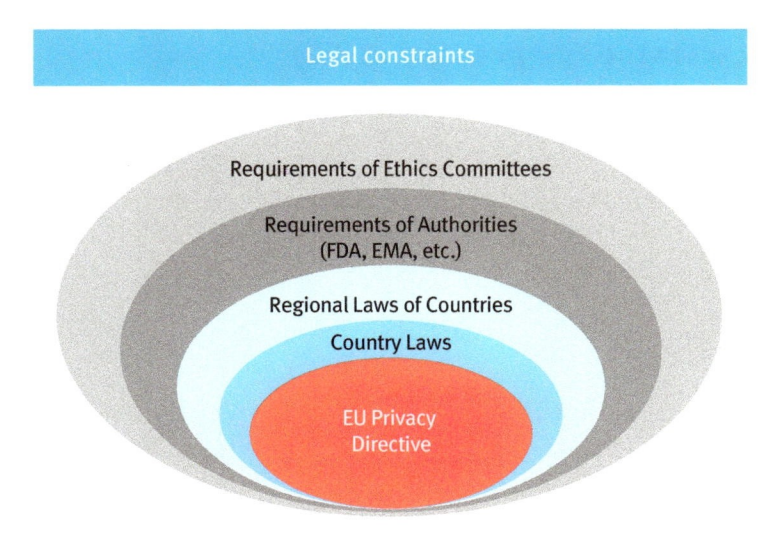

Fig. 10.1 Legal Constraints

Special requirements of international authorities like FDA, EMA (previously EMEA), or other national institutions must be fulfilled in addition.

Prior to enrolling any patient for a clinical study, the complete study concept must be released by the competent Ethics Committee. There may be some restrictions enforced by these boards, especially when conducting clinical trials with a genetic part or when collecting samples for DNA extraction, designated for long-term storage in a biobank.

All those restrictions must be attached to the related samples/patients and taken into account when planning and performing genetic tests and a common statistical analysis of anonymized clinical and related genetic data.

Essentially, there will arise no problems with respect to data protection as long as personal data are processed within the scope of the EU Privacy Directive. Special measures must be implemented prior to transferring personal data to countries outside the European Union. Under which conditions transfer of personal data to so-called third countries is admissible will be explained in the chapter *"Transfer of Personal Data to Third Countries"*.

A major challenge is the processing of personal data within a multinational company the clinical sites of which are not all located in member states of the European Union. We will provide some information and outline a way to go to this special topic in the chapter *"Binding Corporate Rules"*.

To develop a better feeling of what is meant by data protection, and in which way it has to be implemented, we will provide a brief overview of the history of data protection in the European Union and the U.S. in the following.

10.2 Data Protection in the European Union (EU)

To better understand the legal framework of privacy and data protection of the European Union it is necessary to have a clear understanding of the main legislative terms used in this context, i.e. we should be able to clearly distinguish between
- Regulations,
- Directives,
- Decisions, and
- Recommendations, Opinions.

Respective legal definitions are provided by Article 288 of the Treaty on the Functioning of the European Union (cf. (19)). In general, legal acts published in the Official Journal of the European Union are binding. They enter into force the day following that of its publication.

Regulations
are the most powerful instruments of the European legislative. They do not require an additional adoption process into national laws of the Member States, i.e. a special implementation process is not needed. Regulations are in force immediately after their enactment and override the corresponding national laws, if existing, which themselves must fully reflect the spirit of the respective regulations, but could also go beyond.

Directives
are binding for all Member States with respect to the objectives to be achieved. The implementation path of a directive, i.e. the special way how directive objectives are to be incorporated into national law is left to the national authorities.

Decisions
are entirely binding. Decisions that specify its addressees are binding only on them.

Recommendations and **Opinions**
have only an advisory effect but are not binding.

A more comprehensive guide to terminology, procedures and sources of the European Union is issued by the UK House of Commons, cf. (20).

Privacy and **Data Protection** are two separate fundamental rights, but nevertheless closely related to each other. **Respect for private life** has been established for the first time on an European level with the adoption of the *"Council of Europe Convention for the Protection of Human Rights and Fundamental Freedoms (ECHR)"* on 4th November 1950 at Rome, (cf. (21)) The right to privacy may be described as a right which shall prevent **public authorities** from interfering in privacy and from restricting privacy, unless certain conditions are met (cf. ECHR Article 8, below).

The right to privacy is mainly declared in:

Article 5. Equality between spouses

Article 6. Right to a fair trial

Article 8. Right to respect for private and family life
Everyone has the right to respect for his private and family life, his home and his correspondence. There shall be no interference by a public authority with the exercise of this right except such as is in accordance with the law and is necessary in a democratic society in the interests of national security, public safety or the economic well-being of the country, for the prevention of disorder or crime, for the protection of health or morals, or for the protection of the rights and freedoms of others.

Article 9 . Freedom of thought, conscience and religion
Everyone has the right to freedom of thought, conscience and religion; this right includes freedom to change his religion or belief and freedom, either alone or in community with others and in public or private, to manifest his religion or belief, in worship, teaching, practice and observance.

Due to the rapid development of new communication techniques and the resulting new possibilities of data processing and surveillance the right to **data protection** was introduced in 1981.

Data protection principles stipulated conditions for a legitimate and lawful processing of personal data. The "*Convention for the Protection of Individuals with Regard to Automatic Processing of Personal Data, often referred to as Convention 108 (ETS 108)*", was adopted by the Council of Europe on 28th January 1981.

The protection of personal data, granted to an individual as a separate right, was guaranteed for the first time on 28 January 1981 at Strasbourg.

Moreover, Convention 108 is the first legally binding international instrument that has been adopted in the field of data protection.

The right to privacy is emphasized in the preamble of Convention 108,

Preamble
< >
Considering that it is desirable to extend the safeguards for everyone's rights and fundamental freedoms, and in particular the right to the **respect for privacy**, taking account of the increasing flow across frontiers of personal data undergoing automatic processing;
Reaffirming at the same time their commitment to freedom of information regardless of frontiers;
Recognising that it is necessary to reconcile the fundamental values of the **respect for privacy** and the free flow of information between peoples,

and object and purpose of the Convention 108 are declared in its Article 1

Article 1 – Object and purpose
The purpose of this convention is to secure in the territory of each Party for every individual, whatever his nationality or residence, respect for his rights and fundamental freedoms, and in particular his **right to privacy**, with regard to automatic processing of personal data relating to him ("data protection").

Article 3 sets the scope of the Convention to personal data in the public **and** private sector:

Article 3 – Scope
1   The Parties undertake to apply this convention to automated personal data files and automatic processing of personal data in the public and private sectors.

Basic principles for data protection are outlined in Chapter II, and principles for transborder data flows are provided in Chapter III.

On 23rd September 1980, the Organization for Economic Co-operation and Development (OECD) released the "*Guidelines on the Protection of Privacy and Transborder Flows of Personal Data*", which urged its members to implement measures for the protection of personal information.

The Guidelines have been supplemented by an Explanatory Memorandum. In Part Two – *Basic Principles of National Application* – of this memorandum, basic principles like consent, lawfulness and fairness of collection, data quality, purpose of use, disclosure of results, physical security, and openness have been specified.

Collection Limitation Principle
7. There should be limits to the collection of personal data and any such data should be obtained by lawful and fair means and, where appropriate, with the knowledge or consent of the data subject.

Data Quality Principle
8. Personal data should be relevant to the purposes for which they are to be used, and, to the extent necessary for those purposes, should be accurate, complete and kept up-to-date.

Purpose Specification Principle
9. The purposes for which personal data are collected should be specified not later than at the time of data collection and the subsequent use limited to the fulfilment of those purposes or such others as are not incompatible with those purposes and as are specified on each occasion of change of purpose.

Use Limitation Principle
10. Personal data should not be disclosed, made available or otherwise used for purposes other than those specified in accordance with Paragraph 9 except:
    a) with the consent of the data subject; or
    b) by the authority of law.

Security Safeguards Principle
11. Personal data should be protected by reasonable security safeguards against such risks as loss or unauthorised access, destruction, use, modification or disclosure of data.

Openness Principle
12. There should be a general policy of openness about developments, practices and policies with respect to personal data. Means should be readily available of establishing the existence and nature of personal data, and the main purposes of their use, as well as the identity and usual residence of the data controller.

The OECD Guidelines defines personal data as follows:

"*personal data*" *means any information relating to an identified or identifiable individual (data subject).*

A more detailed definition of what is meant by identified or identifiable has not been given. In addition, in contrast to existing international data protection standards, the

OECD Guidelines do not specify particular data protection measures for personal data in the health information sector.

Respect for private and family life and protection of personal data have been judged as closely related and have been declared as separate fundamental rights in Articles 7 and 8 of the EU Charter of Fundamental Rights (cf. (22)), adopted on December 18, 2000 and re-affirmed on December 14, 2007.

> **Article 7**
> **Respect for private and family life**
> Everyone has the right to respect for his or her private and family life, home and communications.
> **Article 8**
> **Protection of personal data**
> 1. Everyone has the right to the protection of personal data concerning him or her.
> 2. Such data must be processed fairly for specified purposes and on the basis of the consent of the person concerned or some other legitimate basis laid down by law. Everyone has the right of access to data which has been collected concerning him or her, and the right to have it rectified.
> 3. Compliance with these rules shall be subject to control by an independent authority.

As outlined above, respect for private life has been ensured at European level since the adoption of the Council of Europe Convention for the Protection of Human Rights and Fundamental Freedoms (ECHR) in 1950 (cf. (21)).

During the next two decades information and communication technologies were characterized by rapid new developments which on the one hand made the daily life of citizens easier with respect to communication, but on the other hand provided also more sophisticated possibilities of surveillance.

The legislation implemented so far did no longer reflect the state of the art. An adaptation and especially expansion of the scope of data protection regulations was perceived as absolutely necessary.

The term **private life** as defined in the ECHR some decades ago had become too restrictive and did mainly cover the protection against possible interferences by public authorities; protection against interferences by private organizations, e.g. companies, had not been taken into account so far.

Starting with Convention 108 as the first legally binding international instrument in the field of data protection, several recommendations covering the distinct aspects of data protection have been adopted by the Committee of Ministers since.

- **Recommendation No.R (81) 1** 1981, Jan 23
  on regulations for automated medical data banks
  Remark: in 1997 replaced by Recommendation No. R(97) 5 including the Explanatory Memorandum
- **Recommendation No.R (83) 10** 1983, Sep 23
  on the protection of personal data used for scientific research and statistics

Explanatory Memorandum
Remark: in 1997 replaced by Recommendation No. R(97) 18 with respect to statistics
- **Recommendation No.R (85) 20**   1985, Oct 25
  on the protection of personal data used for the purposes of direct marketing
  Explanatory Memorandum
- **Recommendation No.R (86) 1**   1986, Jan 23
  on the protection of personal data for social security purposes
  Explanatory Memorandum
- **Recommendation No.R (87) 15**   1987, Sep 17
  regulating the use of personal data in the police sector
  Evaluation reports of the Recommendation
- **Recommendation No. R (89) 2**   1989, Jan 18
  on the protection of personal data used for employment purposes
  Explanatory Memorandum
- **Recommendation No. R (90) 19**   1990, Sep 13
  on the protection of personal data used for payment and other operations
  Explanatory Memorandum
- **Recommendation No. R (91) 10**   1991, Sep 9
  on the communication to third parties of personal data held by public bodies
  Explanatory Memorandum
- **Recommendation No. R (92) 3**   1992, Feb 10
  on Genetic Testing and Screening for Health Care Purposes
- **Recommendation No. R (92) 1**   1992, Feb 10
  on the Use of Analysis of Deoxyribonucleic Acid (DNA) Within the Framework of the Criminal Justice System.
- **Recommendation No. R (95) 4**   1995, Feb 7
  on the protection of personal data in the area of telecommunication services, with particular reference to telephone services
  Explanatory Memorandum
- **Recommendation No. R (97) 5**   1997, Feb 13
  on the protection of medical data
  Explanatory Memorandum
- **Convention on Human Rights and Biomedicine**   1997, Apr 4
  Convention for the Protection of Human Rights and Dignity of the Human Being with Regard to the Application of Biology and Medicine, European Treaty Series – No. 164
- **Recommendation No. R (97) 18**   1997, Sep 30
  on the protection of personal data collected and processed for statistical purposes
  Explanatory Memorandum
- **Recommendation No. R (99) 5**   1999, Feb 23
  for the protection of privacy on the Internet

- **Recommendation No. R (2002) 9** 2002, Sep 18
  on the protection of personal data collected and processed for insurance purposes
  Explanatory Memorandum
- **Recommendation Rec(2006) 4** 2006, Mar 15
  on Research on Biological Materials of Human Origin

In the 1990s, national laws regulating the protection of personal data were not harmonized across the EU Member States, although based on the same principles as issued by the respective COE recommendations and treaties.

The increasing necessity for harmonization of data protection regulations, mainly triggered by economic reasons and new developments in the information and communication area, did finally result in the formulation and subsequent adoption of *"DIRECTIVE 95/46/EC of the European Parliament and of the Council of 24 October 1995 on the protection of individuals with regard to the processing of personal data and on the free movement of such data"*.

- **Directive 95/46/EC** is usually referred to as the **EU Privacy Directive**

It is the central pillar of legislation on the protection of personal data in Europe and applies to the private as well as the public sector.

Nevertheless, the transfer of personal data in the course of judicial and police co-operation activities as specified within *"TITLE V – Provisions on a common foreign and security policy"*, and *"TITLE VI – Provisions on police and judicial cooperation in criminal matters"* of the Treaty on European Union is not covered by the EU Privacy Directive. A regulation for this special purpose has been adopted only in late 2008.

EU Member States are obliged to bring their national laws into conformity with the principles of the EU Privacy Directive within 3 years of its adoption. The respective country laws may have even stronger conditions under which the processing of personal data is lawful, as stated in chapter II of the Directive.

CHAPTER II
GENERAL RULES ON THE LAWFULNESS OF THE PROCESSING OF PERSONAL DATA
Article 5
Member States shall, within the limits of the provisions of this Chapter, determine more precisely the conditions under which the processing of personal data is lawful

The Directive 95/46/EC provides in its article 28 for each Member State to establish one or more public authorities which are responsible for monitoring its local – i.e. in the respective country – implementation.

Article 28 – Supervisory authority
1. Each Member State shall provide that one or more public authorities are responsible for monitoring the application within its territory of the provisions adopted by the Member States pursuant to this Directive. These authorities shall act with complete independence in exercising the functions entrusted to them.

2. Each Member State shall provide that the supervisory authorities are consulted when drawing up administrative measures or regulations relating to the protection of individuals' rights and freedoms with regard to the processing of personal data.

In Article 29 of the Directive 95/46/EC the so-called **Working Party** has been established. The Working Party, usually referred to as **Article 29 Working Party,** is understood to be the independent EU Advisory Body on Data Protection and Privacy. Its special tasks are depicted in Article 30 of Directive 95/46/EC (cf. (23)), in Article 14 of Directive 97/66/EC (cf. (45)), and in Article 15 of Directive 2002/58/EC.

Its rules of procedure, essentially implied by the EU Privacy Directive, has been issued on 18 February 2008 in *"Working Party on the Protection of Individuals with Regard to the Processing of Personal Data – Rules of Procedure"*.

Article 2 provides information on how the Article 29 Working Party is composed. Members of the Article 29 Working Party are consequently representatives of the national data protection authorities (DPA) – usually the national Data Protection Officer – of the currently 28 EU Member States, the European Data Protection Supervisor (EDPS) and the European Commission.

Membership of the Working Party
Article 2
1. The Working Party shall be composed of a representative of the supervisory authority or authorities designated by each Member State, a representative of the European Data Protection Supervisor and a representative of the European Commission. [Art. 29(2)]
2. Each member of the Working Party shall be designated by the institution, authority or authorities which he represents. Where a Member State has designated more than one supervisory authority, they shall nominate a joint representative. [Art. 29(2)]
3. The authorities and institutions mentioned in the above paragraphs shall designate an alternate according to the same procedures. A second alternate may be designated if needed.

Remark: *The quotations in brackets are references to the respective articles of the EU Privacy Directive.*

Status and tasks of the Working Party as an advisory board have been outlined in Article 1 as follows:

Article 1
1. The Working Party shall have advisory status and act independently. [Art. 29(1)]
2. The Working Party shall:
   (a) examine any question covering the application of the national measures adopted under this Directive in order to contribute to the uniform application of such measures;
   (b) give the Commission an opinion on the level of protection in the Community and in third countries;
   (c) advise the Commission on any proposed amendment of this Directive, on any additional or specific measures to safeguard the rights and freedoms of natural persons with regard to the processing of personal data and on any other proposed Community measures affecting such rights and freedoms;
   (d) give an opinion on codes of conduct drawn up at Community level. [Art. 30(1)]

3. If the Working Party finds that divergences likely to affect the equivalence of protection for persons with regard to the processing of personal data in the Community are arising between the laws or practices of Member States, it shall inform the Commission accordingly. [Art. 30(2)]
4. The Working Party may, on its own initiative, make recommendations on all matters relating to the protection of persons with regard to the processing of personal data in the Community.[Art. 30(3)]

Remark: *The quotations in brackets are again references to the respective articles of the EU Privacy Directive.*

The Article 29 Working Party issued from its very beginning numerous opinions to data protection issues. This includes but is not limited to the concept of personal data (cf. WP136) and the processing of personal data relating to health in electronic health records (EHR) (cf. WP131), Genome Issue (cf. WP34), and Genetic Data (cf. WP91).

An excerpt of the Article 29 Working Party Documents covering in particular data protection issues in the health sector and in the electronic communications sector is given below:

- **WP4** 1997, Jun 26
  ARTICLE 29 – Data Protection Working Party on the Protection of Individuals With Regard to the Processing of Personal Data
  First Orientations on Transfers of Personal Data to Third Countries – Possible Ways Forward in Assessing Adequacy
- **WP34** 2000, Jul 13
  ARTICLE 29 – Data Protection Working Party – Opinion 6/2000 on the Genome Issue
- **WP80** 2003, Aug 1
  ARTICLE 29 – Data Protection Working Party – Working document on biometrics
- **WP91** 2004, Mar 17
  ARTICLE 29 – Data Protection Working Party – Working Document on Genetic Data
- **WP114** 2005, Nov 25
  ARTICLE 29 – Data Protection Working Party – Working document on a common interpretation of Article 26(1) of Directive 95/46/EC of 24 October 1995
- **WP131** 2007, Feb 15
  ARTICLE 29 – Data Protection Working Party – Working Document on the processing of personal data relating to health in electronic health records (EHR)
- **WP133** 2007, Jan 10
  ARTICLE 29 – Data Protection Working Party – Recommendation 1/2007 on the Standard Application for Approval of Binding Corporate Rules for the Transfer of Personal Data

- **WP136**   2007, Jun 20
ARTICLE 29 – Data Protection Working Party – Opinion 4/2007 on the concept of personal data
- **WP159**   2009, Feb 10
ARTICLE 29 – Data Protection Working Party – Opinion 1/2009 on the proposals amending Directive 2002/58/EC on privacy and electronic communications (e-Privacy Directive)
- **WP161**   2009, Mar 5
ARTICLE 29 – Data Protection Working Party – Opinion 3/2009 on the Draft Commission Decision on standard contractual clauses for the transfer of personal data to processors established in third countries, under Directive 95/46/EC *(data controller to data processor)*
- **WP165**   2009, Dec 1
ARTICLE 29 – Data Protection Working Party – Opinion 6/2009 on the level of protection of personal data in Israel
- **WP169**   2010, Feb 16
ARTICLE 29 – Data Protection Working Party – Opinion 1/2010 on the concepts of "controller" and "processor"
- **WP176**   2010. Jul 12
ARTICLE 29 – Data Protection Working Party – FAQs in order to address some issues raised by the entry into force of the EU Commission Decision 2010/87/EU of 5 February 2010 on standard contractual clauses for the transfer of personal data to processors established in third countries under Directive 95/46/EC
- **WP187**   2011, Jul 13
ARTICLE 29 – Data Protection Working Party – Opinion 15/2011 on the definition of consent
- **WP191**   2012, Mar 23
ARTICLE 29 – Data Protection Working Party – Opinion 01/2012 on the data protection reform proposals
- **WP195**   2012, Jun 6
ARTICLE 29 – Data Protection Working Party – Working Document 02/2012 setting up a table with the elements and principles to be found in Processor Binding Corporate Rules
- **WP195a**   2012, Sep 17
ARTICLE 29 – Data Protection Working Party – Recommendation 1/2012 on the Standard Application form for Approval of Binding Corporate Rules for the Transfer of Personal Data for Processing Activities
- **WP199**   2012, Oct 5
ARTICLE 29 – Data Protection Working Party – Working Document 01/2013, Input on the proposed implementing acts

- **WP200**   2013, Jan 22
  ARTICLE 29 – Data Protection Working Party – Working Document 01/2013, Input on the proposed implementing acts
- **WP204**   2013, Apr 19
  ARTICLE 29 – Data Protection Working Party – Explanatory Document on the Processor Binding Corporate Rules

Two years after the adoption of the EU Privacy Directive, the expansion of data protection regulations to the telecommunication sector has been accomplished with *"DIRECTIVE 97/66/EC OF THE EUROPEAN PARLIAMENT AND OF THE COUNCIL of 15 December 1997 concerning the processing of personal data and the protection of privacy in the telecommunications sector"*.

Object and scope of this directive are outlined in its Article 1 as follows:

Article 1 – Object and scope
1. This Directive provides for the harmonisation of the provisions of the Member States required to ensure an equivalent level of protection of fundamental rights and freedoms, and in particular the right to privacy, with respect to the processing of personal data in the telecommunications sector and to ensure the free movement of such data and of telecommunications equipment and services in the Community.
2. The provisions of this Directive particularise and complement Directive 95/46/EC for the purposes mentioned in paragraph 1. Moreover, they provide for protection of legitimate interests of subscribers who are legal persons.
3. This Directive shall not apply to the activities which fall outside the scope of Community law, such as those provided for by Titles V and VI of the Treaty on European Union, and in any case to activities concerning public security, defence, State security (including the economic well-being of the State when the activities relate to State security matters) and the activities of the State in areas of criminal law.

Further directives in the sector of electronic communications networks with respect to access control, authorization, framework, and universal services have been adopted in March 2002.
- **DIRECTIVE 2002/22/EC (Universal Service Directive)**   2002, Mar 7
  on universal service and users' rights relating to electronic communications networks and services
- **DIRECTIVE 2002/21/EC (Framework Directive)**   2002, Mar 7
  on a common regulatory framework for electronic communications networks and services
- **DIRECTIVE 2002/20/EC (Authorisation Directive)**   2002, Mar 7
  on the authorisation of electronic communications networks and services
- **DIRECTIVE 2002/19/EC (Access Directive)**   2002, Mar 7
  on access to, and interconnection of, electronic communications networks and associated facilities

DIRECTIVE 97/66/EC has been updated to the then actual standards in 2002 as *"DIRECTIVE 2002/-58/EC OF THE EUROPEAN PARLIAMENT AND OF THE COUNCIL of 12 July 2002 concerning the processing of personal data and the protection of privacy in the electronic communications sector (Directive on privacy and electronic communications)"*

DIRECTIVE 2002/58/EC is usually referred to as the EU ePrivacy Directive

---

The **EU Privacy Directive** and the **EU ePrivacy Directive** form a general framework of data protection across all EU Member States. Scope and aim of the EU ePrivacy Directive are defined in its Article 1 as follows:

Article 1 – Scope and aim
1. This Directive harmonises the provisions of the Member States required to ensure an equivalent level of protection of fundamental rights and freedoms, and in particular the right to privacy, with respect to the processing of personal data in the electronic communication sector and to ensure the free movement of such data and of electronic communication equipment and services in the Community.
2. The provisions of this Directive particularise and complement Directive 95/46/EC for the purposes mentioned in paragraph 1. Moreover, they provide for protection of the legitimate interests of subscribers who are legal persons.
3. This Directive shall not apply to activities which fall outside the scope of the Treaty establishing the European Community, such as those covered by Titles V and VI of the Treaty on European Union, and in any case to activities concerning public security, defence, State security (including the economic well-being of the State when the activities relate to State security matters) and the activities of the State in areas of criminal law.

The EU ePrivacy Directive has been amended in March 2006 by *"DIRECTIVE 2006/24/EC OF THE EUROPEAN PARLIAMENT AND OF THE COUNCIL of 15 March 2006 on the retention of data generated or processed in connection with the provision of publicly available electronic communications services or of public communications networks and amending Directive 2002/58/EC"*.

Subject matter and scope of DIRECTIVE 2006/24/EC are depicted in its Article 1 as follows:

Article 1 – Subject matter and scope
1. This Directive aims to harmonise Member States' provisions concerning the obligations of the providers of publicly available electronic communications services or of public communications networks with respect to the retention of certain data which are generated or processed by them, in order to ensure that the data are available for the purpose of the investigation, detection and prosecution of serious crime, as defined by each Member State in its national law.
2. This Directive shall apply to traffic and location data on both legal entities and natural persons and to the related data necessary to identify the subscriber or registered user. It

shall not apply to the content of electronic communications, including information consulted using an electronic communications network.

Nevertheless, sufficient protection of privacy on the level of EC institutions (e.g. EU Commission, EU Parliament) and the EC bodies (European Food Safety Authority and other agencies) could not be realized by the directives already in place.

To close this gap, article 286 of the EC treaty was adopted in *"Regulation (EC) No 45/2001"*

Article 286 EC Treaty
1. From 1 January 1999, Community acts on the protection of individuals with regard to the processing of personal data and the free movement of such data shall apply to the institutions and bodies set up by, or on the basis of, this Treaty.
2. Before the date referred to in paragraph 1, the Council, acting in accordance with the procedure referred to in Article 251, shall establish an **independent supervisory bod**y responsible for monitoring the application of such Community acts to Community institutions and bodies and shall adopt any other relevant provisions as appropriate.

In the *"Regulation (EC) No 45/2001 of the European Parliament and of the Council of 18 December 2000 on the protection of individuals with regard to the processing of personal data by the Community institutions and bodies and on the free movement of such data"* essentially the same rights and obligations as specified in the EU Privacy Directive are set up at the level of the EC institutions and bodies, cf. Article 27 to 33., e.g.

Article 27 – **Prior checking**
1. Processing operations likely to present specific risks to the rights and freedoms of data subjects by virtue of their nature, their scope or their purposes shall be subject to prior checking by the European Data Protection Supervisor.
2. The risks following processing operations are likely to present such:
    (a) processing of data relating to health and to suspected offences, offences, criminal convictions or security measures;
    (b) processing operations intended to evaluate personal aspects relating to the data subject, including his or her ability, efficiency and conduct;

Regulation (EC) No 45/2001 also establishes the European Data Protection Supervisor (EDPS) as an independent supervisory authority which is responsible for monitoring the processing of personal data by the Community institutions and bodies.

Article 1 – **Object of the Regulation**
1. In accordance with this Regulation, the institutions and bodies set up by, or on the basis of, the Treaties establishing the European Communities, hereinafter referred to as 'Community institutions or bodies', shall protect the fundamental rights and freedoms of natural persons, and in particular their right to privacy with respect to the processing of personal data and shall neither restrict nor prohibit the free flow of personal data between themselves or to recipients subject to the national law of the Member States implementing Directive 95/46/EC.

2. The independent supervisory authority established by this Regulation, hereinafter referred to as the **European Data Protection Supervisor**, shall monitor the application of the provisions of this Regulation to all processing operations carried out by a Community institution or body

Although the EU Privacy Directive does not explicitly define what is meant by medical and genetic data, several directives have been adopted so far, providing rules
- to implement good clinical practice in the conduct of clinical trials,

providing standards of quality and safety, including technical requirements
- for the collection, testing, processing, storage and distribution of human blood and blood components,

setting standards of quality and safety, including technical aspects,
- for the donation, procurement, testing, processing, preservation, storage and distribution of human tissues and cells.

The respective directives are listed in the following:
- **DIRECTIVE 2001/20/EC** 2001, Apr 4
  on the approximation of the laws, regulations and administrative provisions of the Member States relating to the implementation of good clinical practice in the conduct of clinical trials on medicinal products for human use
- **DIRECTIVE 2001/83/EC** 2001, Nov 6
  on the Community code relating to medicinal products for human use
- **DIRECTIVE 2002/98/EC** 2003, Jan 27
  setting standards of quality and safety for the collection, testing, processing, storage and distribution of human blood and blood components and amending Directive 2001/83/EC
- **DIRECTIVE 2004/33/EC** 2004, Mar 22
  implementing Directive 2002/98/EC of the European Parliament and of the Council as regards certain technical requirements for blood and blood components (Text with EEA relevance)
- **DIRECTIVE 2004/23/EC** 2004, Mar 31
  on setting standards of quality and safety for the donation, procurement, testing, processing, preservation, storage and distribution of human tissues and cells
- **DIRECTIVE 2006/17/EC** 2006, Feb 8
  implementing Directive 2004/23/EC of the European Parliament and of the Council as regards certain technical requirements for the donation, procurement and testing of human tissues and cells (Text with EEA relevance)
- **DIRECTIVE 2006/86/EC** 2006, Oct 24
  implementing Directive 2004/23/EC of the European Parliament and of the Council as regards traceability requirements, notification of serious adverse

reactions and events and certain technical requirements for the coding, processing, preservation, storage and distribution of human tissues and cells (Text with EEA relevance)

As mentioned before, the EU Privacy Directive does not cover the transfer of personal data in the course of judicial and police cooperation activities. To close this gap in the legal framework, in late 2008 the *"COUNCIL FRAMEWORK DECISION 2008/977/JHA of 27 November 2008 on the protection of personal data processed in the framework of police and judicial cooperation in criminal matters"* was adopted. Purpose and scope of this framework decision are outlined in its Article 1:

Article 1 – Purpose and scope
1. The purpose of this Framework Decision is to ensure a high level of protection of the fundamental rights and freedoms of natural persons, and in particular their right to privacy, with respect to the processing of personal data in the framework of police and judicial cooperation in criminal matters, provided for by Title VI of the Treaty on European Union, while guaranteeing a high level of public safety.

DECISION 2008/977/JHA differs from the EU Privacy Directive in those parts which describe the special terms in this context.

On December 1, 2009 the Treaty of Lisbon entered into force. The Lisbon Treaty *"2008/C 115/-01 Consolidated versions of the Treaty on European Union and the Treaty on the Functioning of the European Union, 9 May 2008"* emphasizes an explicit right to data protection in its Article 16 (cf. (19)):

Article 16
(ex Article 286 TEC)
1. Everyone has the right to the protection of personal data concerning them.
2. The European Parliament and the Council, acting in accordance with the ordinary legislative procedure, shall lay down the rules relating to the protection of individuals with regard to the processing of personal data by Union institutions, bodies, offices and agencies, and by the Member States when carrying out activities which fall within the scope of Union law, and the rules relating to the free movement of such data. Compliance with these rules shall be subject to the control of independent authorities.
The rules adopted on the basis of this Article shall be without prejudice to the specific rules laid down in Article 39 of the Treaty on European Union.

The term "EC Treaty", i.e. the Treaty Establishing the European Community has been renamed to Treaty on the Functioning of the European Union ("TFEU"),(cf. (19)).

On November 9, 2009, the EDPS welcomes the improvements in the revised ePrivacy Directive.

The revised ePrivacy Directive, as amended by the European Parliament and adopted by the Council, must be implemented by the EU Member States within 18 months after the publication date of the amendments in the Official Journal of the

European Union. Bear in mind that only legal acts published in the Official Journal are binding. They enter into force the day following that of its publication.

The new provisions represent essential improvements in the protection of personal data and privacy with respect to activities in online environments. The changes agreed upon include but are not limited to:

- A framework for mandatory notification of personal data breaches. Among other things, the ePrivacy Directive is amended as follows:

    3. In the case of a personal data breach, the provider of publicly available electronic communications services shall, without undue delay, notify the personal data breach to the competent national authority. When the personal data breach is likely to adversely affect the personal data or privacy of a subscriber or individual, the provider shall also notify the subscriber or individual of the breach without undue delay.

- Fortified protection against interception of users' communications using techniques like spyware or cookies. Subscriber, user must have given consent.

Article 5(3) of the ePrivacy Directive will be replaced by the following:

    3. Member States shall ensure that the storing of information, or the gaining of access to information already stored, in the terminal equipment of a subscriber or user is only allowed on condition that the subscriber or user concerned has given his or her consent, having been provided with clear and comprehensive information, in accordance with Directive 95/46/EC, inter alia about the purposes of the processing.
    This shall not prevent any technical storage or access for the sole purpose of carrying out the transmission of a communication over an electronic communications network, or as strictly necessary in order for the provider of an information society service explicitly requested by the subscriber or user to provide the service.

- Initiation of effective legal proceedings against spammers for any person negatively affected by spam, including (ISPs). The following Article 15a will be inserted:

    Implementation and enforcement
    1. Member States shall lay down the rules on penalties, including criminal sanctions where appropriate, applicable to infringements of the national provisions adopted pursuant to this Directive and shall take all measures necessary to ensure that they are implemented. The penalties provided for must be effective, proportionate and dissuasive and may be applied to cover the period of any breach, even where the breach has subsequently been rectified. The Member States shall notify those provisions to the Commission by ...+, and shall notify it without delay of any subsequent amendment affecting them.

- Substantially strengthened enforcement powers for national data protection authorities, including improved means of cross border cooperation. Article 15a as well:

2. Without prejudice to any judicial remedy which might be available, Member States shall ensure that the competent national authority and, where relevant, other national bodies have the power to order the cessation of the infringements referred to in paragraph 1.
3. Member States shall ensure that the competent national authority and, where relevant, other national bodies have the necessary investigative powers and resources, including the power to obtain any relevant information they might need to monitor and enforce national provisions adopted pursuant to this Directive.
4. The relevant national regulatory authorities may adopt measures to ensure effective cross-border cooperation in the enforcement of the national laws adopted pursuant to this Directive and to create harmonised conditions for the provision of services involving cross-border data flows.

10.3. Transfer of Personal Data to Third Countries

Within the European Union (EU) and the European Economic Area (EAA) transfer of personal data is not subjected to any restrictions, because the EU Privacy Directive is legally binding for all Member States of the EU and it also applies to the EAA countries. According to Article 32 of the EU Privacy Directive all EU Member States are obliged to bring their national data

FINAL PROVISIONS
Article 32
1. Member States shall bring into force the laws, regulations and administrative provisions necessary to comply with this Directive at the latest at the end of a period of three years from the date of its adoption.

protection laws in compliance with the EU Privacy Directive within 3 years of its adoption. This obligation implies that the protection of personal data and privacy can be considered as equivalent across all Member States.

Just as a reminder, EU Member States are:

Austria	Germany	Poland
Belgium	Greece	Portugal
Bulgaria	Hungary	Romania
Croatia	Ireland	Slovakia
Cyprus	Italy	Slovenia
Czech Republic	Latvia	Spain
Denmark	Lithuania	Sweden
Estonia	Luxemburg	United Kingdom
Finland	Malta	
France	Netherlands	

And the four EEA member countries are:

Norway   Liechtenstein   Iceland
Switzerland

- All countries not being a member of the EU or the EEA are considered to be third countries.

In the first instance, the provision of personal data from the EU or EAA countries in third countries, either in printed or electronic form is permitted by the EU Privacy Directive, if and only if the respective third countries ensure an adequate level of data protection. Details of the transfer of personal data to third countries are regulated by Article 25 of the EU Privacy Directive.

CHAPTER IV
TRANSFER OF PERSONAL DATA TO THIRD COUNTRIES
Article 25
Principles
1. The Member States shall provide that the transfer to a third country of personal data which are undergoing processing or are intended for processing after transfer may take place only if, without prejudice to compliance with the national provisions adopted pursuant to the other provisions of this Directive, the third country in question ensures an adequate level of protection.
2. The adequacy of the level of protection afforded by a third country shall be assessed in the light of all the circumstances surrounding a data transfer operation or set of data transfer operations; particular consideration shall be given to the nature of the data, the purpose and duration of the proposed processing operation or operations, the country of origin and country of final destination, the rules of law, both general and sectoral, in force in the third country in question and the professional rules and security measures which are complied with in that country.
3. The Member States and the Commission shall inform each other of cases where they consider that a third country does not ensure an adequate level of protection within the meaning of paragraph 2.
4. Where the Commission finds, under the procedure provided for in Article 31 (2), that a third country does not ensure an adequate level of protection within the meaning of paragraph 2 of this Article, Member States shall take the measures necessary to prevent any transfer of data of the same type to the third country in question.
5. At the appropriate time, the Commission shall enter into negotiations with a view to remedying the situation resulting from the finding made pursuant to paragraph 4.
6. The Commission may find, in accordance with the procedure referred to in **Article 31 (2),** that a third country ensures an adequate level of protection within the meaning of paragraph 2 of this Article, by reason of its domestic law or of the international commitments it has entered into, particularly upon conclusion of the negotiations referred to in paragraph 5, for the protection of the private lives and basic freedoms and rights of individuals. Member States shall take the measures necessary to comply with the Commission's decision.

COMMUNITY IMPLEMENTING MEASURES
Article 31
1. The Commission shall be assisted by a committee.
2. Where reference Is made to this Article, Articles 4 and 7 of Decision 1999/468/EC
   (1) shall apply, having regard to the provisions of Article 8 thereof. The period laid down in Article 4(3) of Decision 1999/468/EC shall be set at three months.
3. The Committee shall adopt its rules of procedure.

The Commission has been empowered by the Council and the European Parliament to determine, on the basis of Article 25(6) of the EU Privacy Directive, whether a third country can guarantee an adequate level of data protection based on its domestic data protection law or on special international commitments it has agreed to.

Details of the procedures are outlined in Article 31 (2) of the EU Privacy Directive and in Articles 4 and 7 of the Council Decision 1999/468/EC, as well as in Council Decision 2006/512/EC.

- **COUNCIL DECISION 1999/468/EC** 1999, Jun 28
  laying down the procedures for the exercise of implementing powers conferred on the Commission
- **COUNCIL DECISION 2006/512/EC** 2006, Jul 17
  amending Decision 1999/468/EC laying down the procedures for the exercise of implementing powers conferred on the Commission

More information on the procedure outlined above can be found on the European Commission website *"Commission decisions on the adequacy of the protection of personal data in third countries"*, cf. http://ec.europa.eu/justice/data-protection/data-collection/data-transfer/index_en.htm managed by the Directorate-General for Justice, Freedom and Security of the European Commission.

The data protection laws of a few countries and/or their special international commitments they have agreed to, have been examined by the EU Commission.

A positive decision with respect to a country implies that personal data, being considered in the commission decision document, may flow from the 28 EU countries and 4 EEA member countries to that third country within the existing framework of data protection of that country. The implementation of further safeguards is not necessary.

In addition, the EU Commission has assessed that the level of protection is adequate in some countries if certain conditions are met.

The level of data protection is considered as adequate in the countries listed below.

- **Andorra** 2010, Oct 19
  COMMISSION DECISION of 19 October 2010 pursuant to Directive 95/46/EC of the European Parliament and of the Council on the adequate protection of personal data in Andorra *(notified under document C(2010) 7084)* (Text with EEA relevance) (2010/625/EU)

- **Argentina** 2003, Jun 30
Commission Decision C(2003)1731 final, of 30/06/2003 pursuant to Directive 95/46/EC of the European Parliament and of the Council on the adequate protection of personal data in Argentina (Text with EEA relevance)
- **Australia** 2008, Jun 30
COUNCIL DECISION 2008/651/CFSP/JHA of 30 June 2008 on the signing, on behalf of the European Union, of an Agreement between the European Union and Australia on the processing and transfer of European Unionsourced passenger name record (PNR) data by air carriers to the Australian Customs Service
- **Canada** 2001, Dec 20
Commission Staff Working Document: The application of Commission Decision 2002/2/EC of 20 December 2001 pursuant to Directive 95/46/EC of the European Parliament and of the Council on the adequate protection of personal data provided by the Canadian Personal Information Protection and Electronic Documentation Act, cf. http://ec.europa.eu/justice/policies/privacy/docs/adequacy/canada_st15644_06_en.pdf

4. CONCLUSION
On the basis of the study and other information collected, the Commission services take the view that the Canadian Personal Information and Electronic Documentation Act continues to provide an adequate level of protection of personal data within the meaning of Article 25 of the Directive. The reservation formulated in Article 3 of Decision 2002/-2/EC12 which contains safeguards necessary in case of data transfers to countries outside the European Union is maintained.

- **Canada** 2005, Sep 6
COMMISSION DECISION of 6 September 2005 on the adequate protection of personal data contained in the Passenger Name Record of air passengers transferred to the Canada Border Services Agency (Text with EEA relevance)(2006/253/EC)
- **Faeroe Islands** 2010 March 5
Commission Decision of 5 March 2010 pursuant to Directive 95/46/EC of the European Parliament and of the Council on the adequate protection provided by the Faeroese Act on processing of personal data (notified under document C(2010) 1130)
- **Guernsey** 2003, Nov 21
Commission Decision 2003/821/EC of 21 November 2003 on the adequate protection of personal data in Guernsey (Text with EEA relevance)
- **Guernsey** 2003, Jun 13
WP 79, ARTICLE 29 Data Protection Working Party, Opinion 5/2003 on the level of protection of personal data in Guernsey, adopted on 13 June 2003.
- **State of Israel** 2011, Jan 31
COMMISSION DECISION of 31 January 2011 pursuant to Directive 95/46/EC of the European Parliament and of the Council on the adequate protection of personal

data by the State of Israel with regard to automated processsing of personal data *(notified under document C(2011) 332)* (Text with EEA relevance) (2011/61/EU)
- **Isle of Man** 2004, Apr 28
Commission Decision 2004/411/EC of 28.4.2004 on the adequate protection of personal data in the Isle of Man.
- **Jersey** 2008, May 8
Commission Decision 2008/393/EC of 8 May 2008 pursuant to Directive 95/46/EC of the European Parliament and of the Council on the adequate protection of personal data in Jersey, (Text with EEA relevance).
- **New Zealand** 2012, Dec 19
COMMISSION IMPLEMENTING DECISION of 19 December 2012 pursuant to Directive 95/46/EC of the European Parliament and of the Council on the adequate protection of personal data by New Zealand *(notified under document C(2012) 9557)* (Text with EEA relevance) (2013/65/EU)
- **Switzerland** 2000, Jul 26
Commission Decision 2000/518/EC of 26 July 2000 pursuant to Directive 95/46/EC of the European Parliament and of the Council on the adequate protection of personal data provided in Switzerland (notified under document number C(2000) 2304) (Text with EEA relevance).
- **UY – Eastern Republic of Uruguay** 2012, Aug 21
COMMISSION IMPLEMENTING DECISION of 21 August 2012 pursuant to Directive 95/46/EC of the European Parliament and of the Council on the adequate protection of personal data by the Eastern Republic of Uruguay with regard to automated processing of personal data *(notified under document C(2012) 5704)* (Text with EEA relevance) (2012/484/EU)
- **US – United States –**
 Transfer of Air Passenger Name Record (PNR) Data 2007, Jul 23
COUNCIL DECISION 2007/551/CFSP/JHA of 23 July 2007on the signing, on behalf of the European Union, of an Agreement between the European Union and the United States of America on the processing and transfer of Passenger Name Record (PNR) data by air carriers to the United States Department of Homeland Security (DHS) (2007 PNR Agreement)
- **US – Safe Harbor** 2000, May 16
WP 32, Article 29 Data Protection Working Party, Opinion 4/2000, on the level of protection provided by the "Safe Harbor Principles", Adopted on 16th May 2000. Data protection is considered to be adequate, if the recipient of personal data has agreed to the so-called Safe Harbor principles

For more information see the following EU documents or access directly the *"Commission decisions on the adequacy of the protection of personal data in third countries"* on the European Commission Website via http://ec.europa.eu/justice/data-protection/document/international-transfers/adequacy/index_en.htm

- **COMMISSION DECISION 2000/520/EC** 2000, Jul 26
  of 26 July 2000 pursuant to Directive 95/46/EC of the European Parliament and of the Council on the adequacy of the protection provided by the safe harbour privacy principles and related frequently asked questions issued by the US Department of Commerce (notified under document number C(2000) 2441), (Text with EEA relevance)
- **COMMISSION DECISION** 2000, Jul 27
  of 27 July 2000 pursuant to Directive 95/46/EC of the European Parliament and of the Council on the adequacy of the protection provided by the Safe Harbor Privacy Principles and related Frequently Asked Questions issued by the US Department of Commerce (Text with EEA relevance)
- **COMMISSION DECISION 2002/16/EC** 2001, Dec 27
  on standard contractual clauses for the transfer of personal data to processors established in third countries, under Directive 95/46/EC (notified under document number C(2001) *4540)* (Text with EEA relevance)
- **COMMISSION STAFF WORKING DOCUMENT** 2004, Oct 10
  The implementation of Commission Decision 520/2000/EC on the adequate protection of personal data provided by the Safe Harbour privacy Principles and related Frequently Asked Questions issued by the US Department of Commerce 20.10.2004 SEC (2004) 1323

The U.S. Department of Commerce's International Trade Administration manages the website *Export.gov* together with the 19 Federal Agencies, cf. http://www.export.gov/safeharbor/index.asp, in order to assist American companies to make use of the Safe Harbor framework.

Nevertheless, there exist situations that require a data transfer to third countries although an appropriate level of data protection has never been assessed before.

The legal background for those derogations from the preferred data transfer is given by article 26 of the EU Privacy Directive.

Article 26
Derogations
1. By way of derogation from Article 25 and save where otherwise provided by domestic law governing particular cases, Member States shall provide that a transfer or a set of transfers of personal data to a third country which does not ensure an adequate level of protection within the meaning of Article 25 (2) may take place on condition that:
(a) the data subject has given his consent unambiguously to the proposed transfer; or
(b) the transfer is necessary for the performance of a contract between the data subject and the controller or the implementation of pre-contractual measures taken in response to the data subject's request; or
(c) the transfer is necessary for the conclusion or performance of a contract concluded in the interest of the data subject between the controller and a third party; or
(d) the transfer is necessary or legally required on important public interest grounds, or for the establishment, exercise or defence of legal claims; or

(e) the transfer is necessary in order to protect the vital interests of the data subject; or
(f) the transfer is made from a register which according to laws or regulations is intended to provide information to the public and which is open to consultation either by the public in general or by any person who can demonstrate legitimate interest, to the extent that the conditions laid down in law for consultation are fulfilled in the particular case.
2. Without prejudice to paragraph 1, a Member State may authorize a transfer or a set of transfers of personal data to a third country which does not ensure an adequate level of protection within the meaning of Article 25 (2), where the controller adduces adequate safeguards with respect to the protection of the privacy and fundamental rights and freedoms of individuals and as regards the exercise of the corresponding rights; such safeguards may in particular result from appropriate contractual clauses.
4. Where the Commission decides, in accordance with the procedure referred to in Article 31 (2), that certain standard contractual clauses offer sufficient safeguards as required by paragraph 2, Member States shall take the necessary measures to comply with the Commission's decision.

Practically, the controller, usually the sending unit, has three different alternatives to ensure the lawfulness of a respective data transfer:

- implementation of additional measures for privacy and data protection, e.g. by using appropriate contractual clauses or binding corporate rules according to article 26.2.
- Adoption of the standard contractual clauses (SCC) of the Commission according to article 26.4.
- Reference to one of the six derogations outlined in article 26.1(a) to (e), if adequate.

Standard Contractual Clauses for controller to controller data transfer are provided by COMMISSION DECISION 2001/497/EC, and an alternative set of Standard Contractual Clauses for controller to controller data transfer has been provided by COMMISSION DECISION 2004/915/EC.

Standard Contractual Clauses for controller to processor data transfer has been issued with COMMISSION DECISION 2002/16/EC.

The new COMMISSION DECISION 2010/87/EU covers now the controller to processor data transfer including the expansion of processing activities to contracted subprocessors at the processors site.

Detailed information is available by the following documents:

- **WP12** 1998, Jul 24
  ARTICLE 29 – Data Protection Working Party – Working Document Transfers of personal data to third countries: Applying Articles 25 and 26 of the EU data protection directive
- **COMMISSION DECISION 2001/497/EC** 2001, Jun 15
  of 15 June 2001 on standard contractual clauses for the transfer of personal data to third countries, under Directive 95/46/EC, (Text with EEA relevance)

- **COMMISSION DECISION 2002/16/EC** 2001, Dec 27
  of 27 December 2001 on standard contractual clauses for the transfer of personal data to processors established in third countries, under Directive 95/46/EC *(notified under document number C(2001) 4540)* (Text with EEA relevance)
- **COMMISSION DECISION 2004/915/EC** 2004, Dec 27
  of 27 December 2004 amending Decision 2001/497/EC as regards the introduction of an alternative set of standard contractual clauses for the transfer of personal data to third countries, (Text with EEA relevance)
- **COMMISSION STAFF WORKING DOCUMENT** 2006, Jan 20
  on the implementation of the Commission decisions on standard contractual clauses for the transfer of personal data to third countries (2001/497/EC and 2002/16/EC)
- Frequently Asked Questions Relating to Transfers 2009
  of Personal Data from the EU/EEA to Third Countries
- **COMMISSION DECISION 2010/87/EU** 2010, Feb 5
  of 5 February 2010 on standard contractual clauses for the transfer of personal data to processors established in third countries under Directive 95/46/EC of the European Parliament and of the Council *(notified under document C(2010) 593)* (Text with EEA relevance)

On March 17, 2009 the Data Protection Unit of the Directorate-General for Justice, Freedom and Security at the European Commission has published on its website answers to *"Frequently Asked Questions Relating to Transfers of Personal Data From the EU/EEA to Third Countries"*.

Answers to these FAQs should help to improve the understanding of the legal framework of the EU with respect to the transfer to third countries of personal data processed in the EU/EEA countries. In particular, the abovementioned document provides an itemized description of a "Step by step decision-making process" that should be passed prior to transferring any personal data.

10.4 Binding Corporate Rules

To facilitate the international transfer of personal data between sites of multinational companies the so-called **Binding Corporate Rules (BCRs)** have been set up,

whereas

BCRs are a legal tool to be used by multinational companies to guarantee an adequate level of protection for the transfers of personal data from a company site located in a country of the EU or the European Economic Area (EEA) to a company site located in a third country (Fig. 10.2)

Basically, making use of BCRs requires the approval of each of the EU or EEA data protection authorities from whose area of authorization data are to be transferred.

In WP74 basic requirements for binding corporate rules have been defined.

In section 5, *"Delivering Compliance and Guaranteeing Enforcement"*, topics like Provisions guaranteeing a good level of compliance, Audits, Complaint handling, the duty of co-operation with data protection authorities, Liability – General right to obtain redress and compensation where appropriate, Rules on liability –, Rules on jurisdiction, and Transparency issues have been addressed.

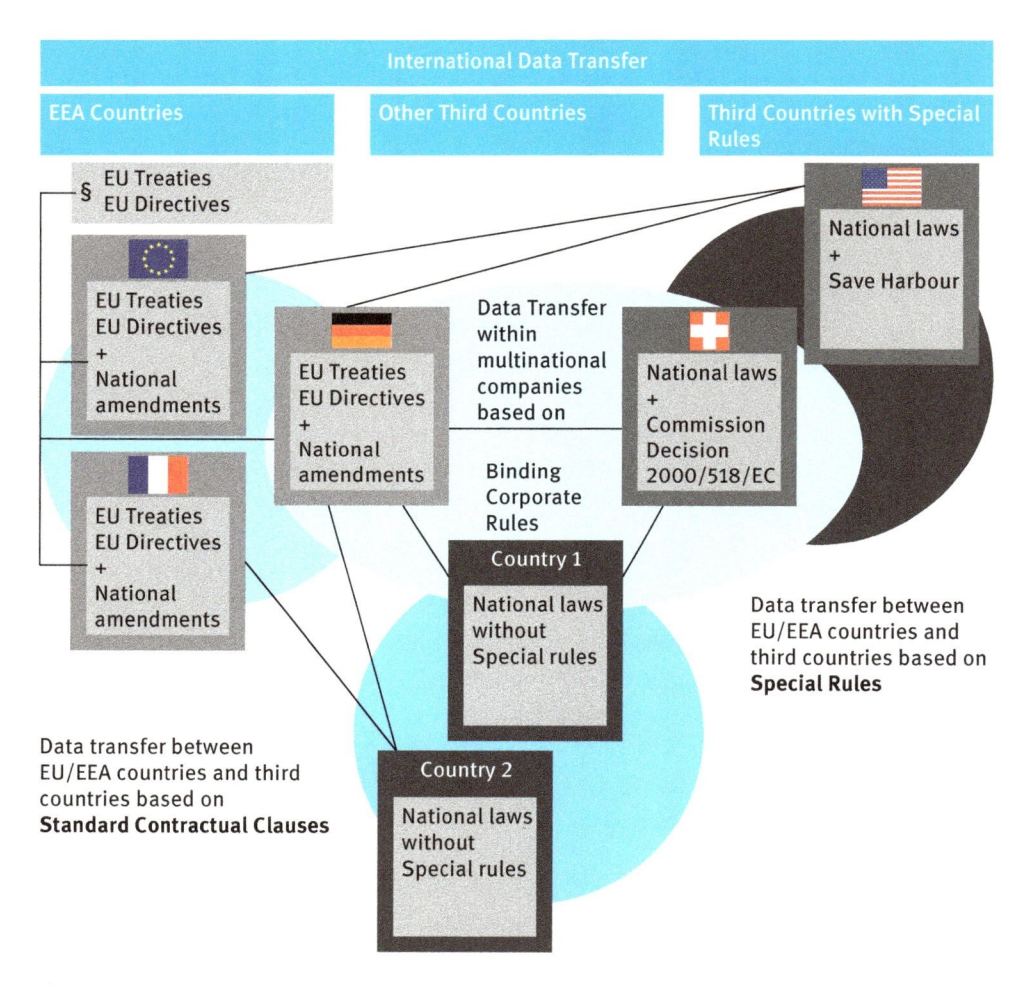

Fig. 10.2 International Data Transfer

In between, the Article 29 Working Party has adopted a number of documents to guide companies interested in using this tool:

A model checklist application for approval of Binding Corporate Rules has been provided by Working Document WP108, adopted on April 14, 2005, and answers to

Frequently Asked Questions (FAQs) related to Binding Corporate Rules have been issued with Working Document WP155rev.04 on April 8, 2009.

An overview of binding corporate rules can be found on the European Commission website, Justice via

http://ec.europa.eu/justice/data-protection/document/international-transfers/binding-corporate-rules/index_en.htm

National filing requirements for authorization of transfers on the basis of BCRs can be accessed via

http://ec.europa.eu/justice/data-protection/document/international-transfers/files/table_nat_admin_req_en.pdf

More detailed information is available in the following documents:

- **WP12** 1998, Jul 24
  ARTICLE 29 – Data Protection Working Party – Working Document Transfers of personal data to third countries: Applying Articles 25 and 26 of the EU data protection directive
- **WP74** 2003, Jun 3
  ARTICLE 29 – Data Protection Working Party – Working Document Transfers of personal data to third countries: Applying Article 26 (2) of the EU Data Protection Directive to Binding Corporate Rules for International Data Transfers
- **WP107** 2005, Apr 14
  ARTICLE 29 – Data Protection Working Party – Working Document Setting Forth a Co-Operation Procedure for Issuing Common Opinions on Adequate Safeguards Resulting From "Binding Corporate Rules"
- **WP108** 2005, Apr 14
  ARTICLE 29 – Data Protection Working Party – Working Document Establishing a Model Checklist Application for Approval of Binding Corporate Rules
- **WP133** 2007, Jan 10
  ARTICLE 29 – Data Protection Working Party – Recommendation 1/2007 on the Standard Application for Approval of Binding Corporate Rules for the Transfer of Personal Data
- **WP153** 2008, Jun 24
  ARTICLE 29 – Data Protection Working Party – Working Document setting up a table with the elements and principles to be found in Binding Corporate Rules
- **WP154** 2008, Jun 24
  ARTICLE 29 – Data Protection Working Party – Working Document Setting up a framework for the structure of Binding Corporate Rules, Adopted on 24 June 2008
- Frequently Asked Questions Relating to Transfers 2009
  of Personal Data from the EU/EEA to Third Countries

- **WP155rev.04**   2009, Apr 8
  ARTICLE 29 – Data Protection Working Party – Working Document on Frequently Asked Questions (FAQs) related to Binding Corporate Rules, Adopted on 24 June 2008, As last Revised and adopted on 8 April 2009
- **WP195a**   2012, Sep 17
  ARTICLE 29 – Data Protection Working Party – Recommendation 1/2012 on the Standard Application form for Approval of Binding Corporate Rules for the Transfer of Personal Data for Processing Activities

10.5. Data Protection in the United States (U.S.) – a Brief History

The following chapter provides a rough survey of some milestones in the United States' history of privacy and data protection.

Prior to going into more details there are some basic administrative facts you should know:
- The rules of the U.S. Food and Drug Administration (FDA) are published in Title 21 of the Code of Federal Regulations (CFR).
- The statutes of the U.S. Public Health Service (PHS) are published in Title 45 of the CFR.

Unlike in Europe, there is no single law in the United States that comprehensively governs privacy and data protection. The United States have mainly regulated the treatment of personal data held by the federal government and its entities, and these regulations are not perceived as an omnibus legislation but moreover as group (institution) or issue specific regulations.

A first corner stone in the U.S. history of data protection is the **Privacy Act of 1974**, 5 U.S.C. § 552a, Public Law No. 93-579, (Dec. 31, 1974), a law that establishes control mechanisms with respect to the collection, use, and disclosure of personal information performed by the federal government. The Privacy Act of 1974 also provides safeguards for privacy rights. Nevertheless this law revealed serious weaknesses. Among other things
- It exclusively covers personal data held by the federal government, it does not cover personal information held by other entities different from the federal government.

> **cf. Section 2 (a)**
> (4) the right to privacy is a personal and fundamental right protected by the Constitution of the United States; and
> (5) in order to protect the privacy of individuals identified in information systems maintained by Federal agencies, it is necessary and proper for the Congress to regulate the collection, maintenance, use, and dissemination of information by such agencies

- It covers only data about U.S. citizens and aliens permanently residing in the U.S., but not data about citizens of other countries.

    cf. Section 3, (a) Definitions
    (2) the term "individual" means a citizen of the United States or an alien lawfully admitted for permanent residence;

- Its protections do not continue after the death of the data subject.
- Its "routine use" provision is not very stringent.

    (b) CONDITIONS OF DISCLOSURE
    No agency shall disclose any record which is contained in a system of records by any means of communication to any person, or to another agency, except pursuant to a written request by, or with the prior written consent of, the individual to whom the record pertains, unless disclosure of the record would be
    (1) to those officers and employees of the agency which maintains the record who have a need for the record in the performance of their duties;
    etc ...

On July 12, 1974, a basic but big legislative step concerning human subjects involved in research projects has been done; the Congress passed the National Research Act (Public Law. 93-348), by which the establishment of Institutional Review Boards (IRB) to review federal funded research projects has been authorized, so far a voluntary measure only. The National Research Act also leads to the appointment of the National Commission for the Protection of Human Subjects of Biomedical and Behavioral Research. This commission compiled reports with respect to the research with human subjects, including recommendations to the then Department of Health, Education, and Welfare (DHEW), in the meantime renamed the Department of Health and Human Services (DHHS).

The best-known of these reports is "The Belmont Report: Ethical Principles and Guidelines for the Protection of Human Subjects of Research" of April 18, 1979. The basic principles of the Belmont Report are provided in three different sections:
- Boundaries Between Practice and Research,
- Basic Ethical Principles, and
- Applications.

Section B itself points out three main ethical principles:

1. Respect for Persons.
Respect for persons incorporates at least two ethical convictions: first, that individuals should be treated as autonomous agents, and second, that persons with diminished autonomy are entitled to protection. The principle of respect for persons thus divides into two separate moral requirements: the requirement to acknowledge autonomy and the requirement to protect those with diminished autonomy......

2. Beneficence.
Persons are treated in an ethical manner not only by respecting their decisions and protecting them from harm, but also by making efforts to secure their well being. Such treatment falls under the principle of beneficence. The term "beneficence" is often understood to cover acts of kindness or charity that go beyond strict obligation. In this document, beneficence is understood in a stronger sense, as an obligation. Two general rules have been formulated as complementary expressions of beneficent actions in this sense: (1) do not harm and (2) maximize possible benefits and minimize possible harms......

3. Justice.
Who ought to receive the benefits of research and bear its burdens? This is a question of justice, in the sense of "fairness in distribution" or "what is deserved." An injustice occurs when some benefit to which a person is entitled is denied without good reason or when some burden is imposed unduly. Another way of conceiving the principle of justice is that equals ought to be treated equally. However, this statement requires explication. Who is equal and who is unequal? What considerations justify departure from equal distribution? Almost all commentators allow that distinctions based on experience, age, deprivation, competence, merit and position do sometimes constitute criteria justifying differential treatment for certain purposes. It is necessary, then, to explain in what respects people should be treated equally. There are several widely accepted formulations of just ways to distribute burdens and benefits. Each formulation mentions some relevant property on the basis of which burdens and benefits should be distributed. These formulations are

(1) to each person an equal share,
(2) to each person according to individual need,
(3) to each person according to individual effort,
(4) to each person according to societal contribution, and
(5) to each person according to merit.

Although never officially adopted, the Belmont Report may be considered as the main ethical framework for the protection of human subjects involved in research in the U.S.. The basic ethical principles outlined in the Belmont Report have triggered several laws prepared by DHHS, e.g.
- 21 CFR Part 50 and 45 CFR Part 46, Protection of Human Subjects, and
- 21 CFR Part 56, Institutional Review Boards.

Institutional Review Boards and the closely related topic informed consent issues are discussed separately in the next chapter. In the Federal Register/Vol. 47, No. 60/ Monday, March 29, 1982, the **DEPARTMENT OF HEALTH AND HUMAN SERVICES** published the report *"Protection of Human Subjects; First Biennial Report on the Adequacy and Uniformity of Federal Rules and Policies, and Their Implementation for the Protection of Human Subjects in Biomedical and Behavioral Research; Report of the President's Commission for the Study of Ethical Problems in Medicine and Biomedical and Behavioral Research."*

On June 18, 1991 these rules have been published as 45 CFR 46, consisting of subparts A, B, C, and D. The DHHS 45 Part 46 regulations are mainly based on principles already outlined in the Belmont Report. They provide a framework for the protection of human subjects involved in DHHS supported biomedical and behavioral research activities. Actual versions of 45 Part 46 regulations are available via the DHHS website http://www.hhs.gov/regulations/, or directly via

http://www.hhs.gov/ohrp/humansubjects/guidance/45cfr46.html.

In 1991 14 further Federal Departments and agencies, listed below, adopted similar rules for the protection of human subjects, identical to subpart A of the DHHS regulation 45 Part 46. This common set of rules is usually referred to as the "**Common Rule**" (cf. (25)).

Regulation Federal Departments/Agencies

7 CFR Part 1c	Department of Agriculture
10 CFR Part 745	Department of Energy
14 CFR Part 1230	National Aeronautics and Space Administration
15 CFR Part 27	Department of Commerce
16 CFR Part 1028	Consumer Product Safety Commission
22 CFR Part 225	International Development Cooperation Agency, Agency for International Development
24 CFR Part 60	Department of Housing and Urban Development
28 CFR Part 46	Department of Justice
32 CFR Part 219	Department of Defense
34 CFR Part 97	Department of Education
38 CFR Part 16	Department of Veterans Affairs
40 CFR Part 26	Environmental Protection Agency
45 CFR Part 690	National Science Foundation
49 CFR Part 11	Department of Transportation

The rapid development of new communication techniques offered new possibilities of electronically transmitting personal health information. The then available legal framework with respect to privacy and protection of personal data seemed to be no longer adequate and therefore required basic enhancements and revisions. As a consequence, the Health Insurance Portability and Accountability Act of 1996 (HIPAA), Public Law 104-191, was enacted on August 21, 1996. Subtitle F, Administrative Simplification, Sections 261 through 264 of HIPAA

SEC. 261. PURPOSE.
It is the purpose of this subtitle to improve the Medicare program under title XVIII of the Social Security Act, the medicaid program under title XIX of such Act, and the efficiency and effectiveness of the health care system, by encouraging the development of a health information system through the establishment of standards and requirements for the electronic transmission of certain health information.
SEC. 262. ADMINISTRATIVE SIMPLIFICATION
SEC. 263. CHANGES IN MEMBERSHIP AND DUTIES OF NATIONAL COMMITTEE ON VITAL AND HEALTH STATISTICS.
SEC. 264. RECOMMENDATIONS WITH RESPECT TO PRIVACY OF CERTAIN HEALTH INFORMATION.

required the DHHS to specify and issue standards for individually identifiable health information, if Congress would not enact privacy legislation within three years of the release of HIPAA.

Because Congress did not enact privacy standards by that deadline, DHHS itself issued Standards for Privacy of Individually Identifiable Health Information in 45 CFR Parts 160 and 164 (**Final Rule**).

These rules also cover information on deceased persons, i.e. the rights to privacy continue after the death of a subject.

The HIPAA Privacy Rule establishes national standards to protect personal health information including individual medical records.

It applies to health plans, health care clearinghouses, and health care providers conducting health care transactions, listed in section 1173(a)(1) of the Health Insurance Portability and Accountability Act of 1996 (HIPAA), electronically.

> "**SEC. 1172.** (a) APPLICABILITY-Any standard adopted under this part shall apply, in whole or in part, to the following persons:
> "(1) A health plan.
> "(2) A health care clearinghouse.
> "(3) A health care provider who transmits any health information in electronic form in connection with a transaction referred to in section 1173(a)(1).

The HIPAA Privacy Rule requires appropriate safeguards to protect the privacy of personal health information.

> (2) SAFEGUARDS.--Each person described in section 1172(a) who maintains or transmits health information shall maintain reasonable and appropriate administrative, technical, and physical safeguards
> (A) to ensure the integrity and confidentiality of the information;
> (B) to protect against any reasonably anticipated
> (i) threats or hazards to the security or integrity of the information; and
> (ii) unauthorized uses or disclosures of the information; and
> (C) otherwise to ensure compliance with this part by the officers and employees of such person.

It also sets standards for the control of protected health information – by setting forth which uses and disclosures are authorized in general, which limitations are to be taken into account – and for the patients' rights on their individual health information.

This includes the patient's rights to examine and obtain a copy of their health records, and to request corrections. The Privacy Rule is issued at 45 CFR Part 160 and Subparts A and E of Part 164. The Electronic Transaction Standards are covered by 45 CFR Part 162

> **Section 164.502(f)—Deceased Individuals**
> We proposed to extend privacy protections to the protected health information of a deceased individual for two years following the date of death. During the two-year time frame, we pro-

posed in the definition of "individual" that the right to control the deceased individual's protected health information would be held by an executor or administrator, or other person (e.g., next of kin) authorized under applicable law to act on behalf of the decedent's estate. The only proposed exception to this standard allowed for uses and disclosures of a decedent's protected health information for research purposes without the authorization of a legal representative and without the Institutional Review Board (IRB) or privacy board approval required (in proposed § 164.510(j)) for most other uses and disclosures for research.

In the final rule (§ 164.502(f)), we modify the standard to extend protection of protected health information about deceased individuals for as long as the covered entity maintains the information. We retain the exception for uses and disclosures for research purposes, now part of § 164.512(i), but also require that the covered entity take certain verification measures prior to release of the decedent's protected health information for such purposes (see §§ 164.514(h) and 164.512(i)(1)(iii)).

We remove from the definition of "individual" the provision related to deceased persons. Instead, we create a standard for "personal representatives" (§ 164.502(g), see discussion below) that requires a covered entity to treat a personal representative of an individual as the individual in certain circumstances, i.e., allows the representative to exercise the rights of the individual. With respect to deceased individuals, the final rule describes when a covered entity must allow a person who otherwise is permitted under applicable law to act with respect to the interest of the decedent or on behalf of the decedent's estate, to make decisions regarding the decedent's protected health information.

The final rule also adds a provision to § 164.512(g), that permits covered entities to disclose protected health information to a funeral director, consistent with applicable law, as necessary to carry out their duties with respect to the decedent. Such disclosures are permitted both after death and in reasonable anticipation of death.

Whereas the Privacy Act of 1974 covers only personal data collected and processed by the federal government, HIPAA broadens the range of covered entities to privately owned companies having their focus on the medical field.

Processing of medical data, i.e. collection, storage, use in general, and also disclosure of those data is subjected to the HIPAA Privacy rules.

A special subset of medical data, generally conceived as being more sensitive than other medical data, are data related to the genetic make-up of individuals, usually denoted as genetic data. Those highly sensitive personal data require a higher level of protection than other personal data.

On May 21, 2008, The Genetic Information Nondiscrimination Act of 2008 (P.L. 110-233, 122 Stat. 881)1, also referred to as GINA, has been signed by the President of the United States. GINA is a new Federal law by which discrimination in health coverage and employment based on genetic information is prohibited (cf. (26)).

On March 24, 2009 the Office of Human Research Protections (OHRP) issued Guidance on the Genetic Information Nondiscrimination Act for Investigators and IRBs (cf. (27)).

On April 6, 2009, the Department of Health and Human Services (DHHS) issued a GINA fact sheet providing information for Researchers and Health Care Professionals, (cf. (28)).

All sections of GINA relating to health coverage will take effect until May 21, 2010 at the latest.

The sections relating to employment are effective since November 21, 2009. For further aspects see also (29), and (30).

11 Informed Consent

The Nuremberg Code of August 1947 defines 10 principles to protect the rights of human subjects that must be met when carrying out medical experiments. This ethical framework in the context of medical research expresses in its first requirement that *"the voluntary consent of the human subject is absolutely essential."*

Although never officially enacted, the Nuremberg Code is being considered as one of the most important basic documents in the development of an ethical framework for medical research. Several other documents like the U.S. *"Belmont Report: Ethical Principles and Guidelines for the Protection of Human Subjects of Research"* of April 18, 1979, or the World Medical Associations' *"Declaration of Helsinki"* of 1964 and the subsequent revisions of it, (cf. (31)), (downloadable from the WMA website) and also regulations like the U.S. 45 CFR 46 take their roots directly or indirectly from the Nuremberg Code.

The *Declaration of Helsinki* defines the basic principles of Informed Consent in its articles 24 and 25 as follows, (cf. (31)).

24. In medical research involving competent human subjects, each potential subject must be adequately informed of the aims, methods, sources of funding, any possible conflicts of interest, institutional affiliations of the researcher, the anticipated benefits and potential risks of the study and the discomfort it may entail, and any other relevant aspects of the study. The potential subject must be informed of the right to refuse to participate in the study or to withdraw consent to participate at any time without reprisal. Special attention should be given to the specific information needs of individual potential subjects as well as to the methods used to deliver the information. After ensuring that the potential subject has understood the information, the physician or another appropriately qualified individual must then seek the potential subject's freely-given informed consent, preferably in writing. If the consent cannot be expressed in writing, the nonwritten consent must be formally documented and witnessed.
25. For medical research using identifiable human material or data, physicians must normally seek consent for the collection, analysis, storage and/or reuse. There may be situations where consent would be impossible or impractical to obtain for such research or would pose a threat to the validity of the research. In such situations the research may be done only after consideration and approval of a research ethics committee.

In principle, data processing with personal data is not allowed and must not be done if an informed consent is missing, i.e. the legitimacy of processing personal data is only given if an informed consent of the respective data subjects has been given.

The EU Privacy Directive (cf. (23)) outlines this basic requirement of an informed consent in more certain terms. More specifically, articles 7 and 8 provide some rules that must be met prior to processing personal data. It is explicitly mentioned that personal data may be processed *"only if the data subject has unambiguously given consent"* subject to an explicit necessary standard.

In its section II – criteria for making data processing legitimate, article 7 – the EU Privacy Directive clearly defines the conditions that must be met prior to processing of personal data.

> **Article 7**
> Member States shall provide that personal data may be processed only if:
> (a) the data subject has unambiguously given his consent; or ...

Section III – special categories of processing, article 8, provides a list of highly sensitive personal data that must not be processed.

> **Article 8:** The Processing of Special Categories of Data
> 1. Member States shall prohibit the processing of personal data revealing racial or ethnic origin, political opinions, religious or philosophical beliefs, trade-union membership, and the processing of data concerning health or sex life.

The definitions used by the EU Privacy Directive are declared in its article 2 and can be also seen in *"Appendix I, EU Privacy Directive – Definitions"*, e.g.

> (h) 'the data subject's **consent**' shall mean any **freely** given **specific** and **informed** indication of his wishes by which the data subject signifies his agreement to personal data relating to him being processed.

Some excerpts from the EU Privacy Directive concerning the area of informed consent are provided in *"Appendix 4, EU Privacy Directive (October 24, 1995)"*.

Subjects taking part in a study should understand all aspects of that study. Single steps of a planned study must be explained in full detail, in an understandable language so that subjects completely comprehend the scenario and perceive themselves as being involved in the study project.

> "Tell me and I forget, show me and I remember, involve me and I understand."
> *Benjamin Franklin*

The *"Convention for the Protection of Human Rights and Dignity of the Human Being with regard to the Application of Biology and Medicine: Convention on Human Rights and Biomedicine, (Oviedo Convention)"*, European Treaty Series – No. 164, 1997, (cf. (32)), emphasizes in its article 5 the necessity of a free informed consent as follows:

> **Chapter II – Consent, Article 5 – General rule**
> An intervention in the health field may only be carried out after the person concerned has given free and informed consent to it. This person shall beforehand be given appropriate information as to the purpose and nature of the intervention as well as on its consequences and risks. The person concerned may freely withdraw consent at any time.

DIRECTIVE 2001/20/EC OF THE EUROPEAN PARLIAMENT AND OF THE COUNCIL of 4 April 2001 on the approximation of the laws, regulations and administrative provisions of the Member States relating to the implementation of good clinical practice in the conduct of clinical trials on medicinal products for human use (cf. (18)) defines informed consent in its *"article 2 Definition (j)"* as follows:

> 'informed consent': decision, which must be written, dated and signed, to take part in a clinical trial, taken freely after being duly informed of its nature, significance, implications and risks and appropriately documented, by any person capable of giving consent or, where the person is not capable of giving consent, by his or her legal representative; if the person concerned is unable to write, oral consent in the presence of at least one witness may be given in exceptional cases, as provided for in national legislation.

Informed Consent issues are discussed in article 4.8 *"Informed Consent of Trial Subjects"* of the ICH – Guideline for Good Clinical Practice, E6(R1) in full detail, (cf. (1)). Article 4.8.10 provides a summary of sections needed in an IC document.

> Both the informed consent discussion and the written informed consent form and any other written information to be provided to subjects should include explanations of the following:
> (a) That the trial involves research.
> (b) The purpose of the trial.
> (c) The trial treatment(s) and the probability for random assignment to each treatment.
> (d) The trial procedures to be followed, including all invasive procedures.
> (e) The subject's responsibilities.
> (f) Those aspects of the trial that are experimental.
> (g) The reasonably foreseeable risks or inconveniences to the subject and, when applicable, to an embryo, fetus, or nursing infant.
> (h) The reasonably expected benefits. When there is no intended clinical benefit to the subject, the subject should be made aware of this.
> (i) The alternative procedure(s) or course(s) of treatment that may be available to the subject, and their important potential benefits and risks.
> (j) The compensation and/or treatment available to the subject in the event of trial-related injury.
> (k) The anticipated prorated payment, if any, to the subject for participating in the trial.
> (l) The anticipated expenses, if any, to the subject for participating in the trial.
> (m) That the subject's participation in the trial is voluntary and that the subject may refuse to participate or withdraw from the trial, at any time, without penalty or loss of benefits to which the subject is otherwise entitled.
> (n) That the monitor(s), the auditor(s), the IRB/IEC, and the regulatory authority(ies) will be granted direct access to the subject's original medical records for verification of clinical trial procedures and/or data, without violating the confidentiality of the subject, to the extent permitted by the applicable laws and regulations and that, by signing a written informed consent form, the subject or the subject's legally acceptable representative is authorizing such access.
> (o) That records identifying the subject will be kept confidential and, to the extent permitted by the applicable laws and/or regulations, will not be made publicly available. If the results of the trial are published, the subject's identity will remain confidential.

(p) That the subject or the subject's legally acceptable representative will be informed in a timely manner if information becomes available that may be relevant to the subject's willingness to continue participation in the trial.
(q) The person(s) to contact for further information regarding the trial and the rights of trial subjects, and whom to contact in the event of trial related injury.
(r) The foreseeable circumstances and/or reasons under which the subject's participation in the trial may be terminated.
(s) The expected duration of the subject's participation in the trial.
(t) The approximate number of subjects involved in the trial.

In the U.S., informed consent issues for research involving human subjects are basically regulated by 14 principles.

For all federal funded research these principles are formulated in the sections
- 46.116 General requirements for informed consent, and
- 46.117 Documentation of informed consent

of Code of Federal Regulations TITLE 45 PUBLIC WELFARE, Department of Health and Human Services, PART 46 PROTECTION OF HUMAN SUBJECTS.

For all research reviewed by the FDA these principles are defined in 21 CFR Part 50, Protection of Human Subjects in "*Subpart B Informed Consent of Human Subjects*", sections 50.20 to 50.27.
- 50.20 General requirements for informed consent.
- 50.21 Effective date.
- 50.23 Exception from general requirements.
- 50.24 Exception from informed consent requirements for emergency research.
- 50.25 Elements of informed consent.
- 50.27 Documentation of informed consent.

The following 8 main principles must be reflected by an informed consent designed for research studies involving human subjects.
(1) Notification that the intended study involves research, including a description of purpose, applied procedures, and expected duration.
(2) Discussion of possible risks or discomforts to the subjects involved.
(3) Description of benefits to the subject and the community.
(4) Explanation of alternative procedures.
(5) Maintenance of confidentiality of collected data.
(6) Availability of treatment in case of injuries.
(7) Contact addresses for answering research related questions.
(8) Statement with respect to voluntariness of participation, including an explanation that a withdrawal from the study is possible at any time without any disadvantage.

Additional 6 sections must be amended if adequate. For detailed information compare the respective sections of 45 CFR 46 (cf. (33)) and 21 CFR 50 (cf. (34)).

William W. Lowrance outlines in his report "Privacy and Health Research, A Report to the U.S. Secretary of Health and Human Services, May 1997" (cf. (42)) some basic ideas in the context of IC. He postulates:
– The ideal is prior, informed, freely granted, specific consent,

while consent is considered to be "free" if the data subject has the possibility
– to refuse his/her consent,
– to withdraw it, or
– to modify the terms and conditions of consent.

W. Lowrance also has discussed the question how broad a consent should be sought for future studies that cannot be specifically anticipated. He made the following statement:

> How meaningful and sufficient is omnibus, indefinite consent?
> Alas, as the ethicist Ruth Faden has rightly lamented:
> As a practical matter, how much moral weight the typical consent to access information can bear is dubious. The **catchall phrases** in the waivers and disclosure statements read and signed by patients and consumers —"Your records will be kept confidential and not be made available, except for statistical purposes," "except for research purposes," and "except for administrative purposes"– **are doubtless not very meaningful to most people.**

Similar considerations can be found in other guidelines and recommendations, too. The ICH – Guideline for Good Clinical Practice, E6(R1), (cf. (1)) expresses this requirement as follows:

> "The language used ... should be as non-technical as practical and should be understandable to the subject".

Regulations in the context of informed consent describe primarily the processing specifics of personal data on the whole. No difference has been made so far between the processing of medical and genetic data. Patients taking part in a clinical study having also a genetic subpart, may freely decide whether to take part also in the genetic subpart or only in the clinical part of the study. A patient decision not to take part in the genetic subpart of a clinical study does not lead to an exclusion of that patient from the whole study in general. The only exception where a patient cannot be included into a respective clinical study are studies running in screening mode. Those studies require provision of genetic information during patients' screening in order to prove the presence of a special genetic make-up defined as inclusion criteria.

Patients taking part in the clinical part as well as in the genetic subpart of a study may freely decide at any time to withdraw from any part/subpart of a study. It is therefore necessary to handle the informed consent approach separately for the clinical part and the genetic subpart of a respective study.

Nevertheless, all features being part of the clinical informed consent are also relevant without any modification or only slightly modified, if adequate, for a genetic informed consent. Some new formulation especially tailored to the processing of genetic samples and data must be amended to the formulations of a genetic informed consent.

A general definition what we should understand by the wording **"Informed Consent"** when conducting pharmacogenetic studies or also clinical studies with a genetic subpart has been given in 2002 by Andersen et al in *"Elements of informed consent for pharmacogenetic research; perspective of the pharmacogenetics working group"*, (cf. (36)); this definition is as follows:

> Informed consent (IC) is the means by which potential research subjects make a judgment about the contribution that their involvement in the research can make, relative to the risks or benefits to them as individuals.

A summary of "Key issues in Informed Consent for pharmacogenomics research" has been also published by Andersen et al on behalf of the Pharmacogenetics Working Group (cf. (36)); more details are provided in Appendix 4.

The Pharmacogenetics Working Group compiled a list of topics to be discussed within a genetic informed consent. We only summarize the main issues related to samples collected during a clinical study with a genetic subpart. All other topics basically reflect the informed consent requirements already known.

A genetic informed consent should provide explanations to the following topics:
- Method of sample collection.
- IC documents used – same IC for the drug trial and for the genetic substudy, or different approaches?
- Participation in main study and/or genetic subpart. Which combinations are possible?
- Archiving of DNA.
- Sample storage: procedures, location, timeframe, etc.
- Data protection measures to guarantee confidentiality.
- Level of sample anonymity: de-identified, anonymized.
- Ownership of the samples.
- Planned use of genetic material: only primary or also secondary use?
- Distribution of genetic material to secondary users.
- Sharing of unintended genetic results.

The Council for International Organizations of Medical Sciences (CIOMS) published in its *"International Ethical Guidelines for Biomedical Research Involving Human Subjects, prepared by the Council for International Organizations of Medical Sciences*

(CIOMS) in collaboration with the World Health Organization (WHO)" of 2002 and in *"Annex 2 to these Guidelines"* of 2005, August 5, (cf. (37) and (38)) a listing of information to be provided prior to signing an informed consent for a research project.

According to these Guidelines information with respect to the following topics must be explained to the data subjects in an understandable language, either orally or in another adequate form, e.g. in writing, prior to asking the data subject to sign an informed consent:

> "Add little to little and there will be a big pile"
> ("Adde parvum parvo magnus acervus erit")
> *Ovid*

- Inclusion criteria for voluntary research, emphasizing that participation is free, and a withdrawal is possible at any time without any personal disadvantages.
- Intended research project, including explanations of statistical study design and unblinding procedures, if adequate, as well as explanations of specified time schedule, duration of studies, planned visits, etc.
- Financial compensation.
- Notification of participants after completion of the study.
- Right to access the personal data.
- Expected risks when participating as well as expected benefits to the participants and the community.
- Posterior official availability of study related products or interventions.
- Alternative treatments, if available.
- Provisions being made to guarantee privacy of subjects and the confidentiality of personal data collected as well as consequences of unforeseeable security breaches.
- Policy with respect to the use of derived genetic data and familial genetic information, including measures being implemented to prevent disclosure of the genetic data to immediate family relatives or to others (e.g. insurance companies or employers) without the explicit consent of the data subject.
- Information with respect to sponsor, investigator and funding of the planned study.
- Use of subject's medical data and of biological samples collected during the study, including the right to refuse storage, and the right to require destruction of collected material.
- Planned development of commercial products from biological samples, and possible benefits for the participants of the study.
- Role of the investigator.
- Free of charge provision of treatment for specified types of research related injury and/or for related complications, including explanation of patient insurance.
- Review and approval of research protocol by competent Ethics Committees.

The International Declaration on Human Genetic Data, adopted unanimously and by acclamation on 16 October 2003 by the 32nd session of the General Conference of UNESCO (cf. (4)) states precisely in its respective articles some main issues in the context of genetic informed consent:

- Article 7: Non-discrimination and non-stigmatization.
- Article 8: Consent.
- Article 9: Withdrawal of consent.
- Article 10: The right to decide whether or not to be informed about research results.
- Article 11: Genetic counseling.
- Article 13: Access.
- Article 14: Privacy and Confidentiality.
- Article 15: Accuracy, reliability, quality and security.
- Article 16: Change of purpose.
- Article 17: Stored biological samples.

Important integral parts of a genetic IC are also statements on how confidentiality and privacy will be maintained and how genetic privacy will be guaranteed.

The special terms used are defined in Article 2 of the declaration, e.g.

Human genetic data:
Information about heritable characteristics of individuals obtained by analysis of nucleic acids or by other scientific analysis.

Consent:
Any freely given specific, informed and express agreement of an individual to his or her genetic data being collected, processed, used and stored.

The "*UNESCO Universal Declaration on Bioethics and Human Rights*" (cf. (39)), adopted by acclamation on 19 October 2005 by the 33rd session of the General Conference of UNESCO requires in its article 6 the agreement of an informed consent for

Any preventive, diagnostic and therapeutic medical intervention
Any scientific research

Consent must be provided in understandable form, so that participants can comprehend it, and a withdrawal of consent must be possible at any time without any disadvantages. If research is carried out on a group of persons, individual consents of all group members are required; a collective group consent or a consent signed by a designated group member is not sufficient.

Human Genetic Examination Act (Genetic Diagnosis Act – GenDG), April 24, 2009 (cf. (40))

Consent
(1) Any genetic examination or analysis may only be conducted, and any genetic sample may only be acquired for such a purpose, after the responsible medical person has received the express, written consent of the subject person, both in regard to the respective genetic examination and genetic sample. The consent stated in the foregoing sentence includes the decision in regard to the scope of the given genetic examination as well as regarding the decisions if, and if so to which extent, the examination results may be disclosed or, as the case may be, destroyed. A person or institution authorized according to § 7 (2) may only conduct any genetic analysis given proof of consent.
(2) The subject person may at any time with future effect revoke his or her permission vis-à-vis the responsible medical person either orally or in writing. Any oral revocation must be immediately documented. The responsible medical person must immediately transmit a copy of the proof of revocation of consent to the person or institution commissioned or authorized according to § 7 (2).

The Seventh Framework Programme for research and technological development (FP7) was the European Union's main instrument for funding research in Europe in the years 2007-2013, providing for its applicants an itemized ethical framework.

Further information with respect to informed consent issues can be found within the FP7 Ethical Guidelines on the CORDIS (**CO**mmunity **R**esearch and **D**evelopment **I**nformation **S**ervice) website.

(cf. http://cordis.europa.eu/fp7/ethics_en.html)

In particular, compare the ethical review in FP7, "Guidance for Applicants, Informed Consent", http://ec.europa.eu/research/participants/data/ref/fp7/89807/informed-consent_en.pdf

FP7 is being succeeded by H2020, "Horizon 2020", the EU Framework Programme for Research and Innovation, planned for the period 2014 – 2020.

(cf. http://ec.europa.eu/programmes/horizon2020/en/)

Recalling the four possible approaches of clinical studies including a genetic part, we recommend to cover these different trial types also with respective distinct genetic informed consents, i.e. we must provide genetic informed consents for
- Screening Mode,
- Prespecified Mode,
- Unspecified Mode, and
- Prespecified and Unspecified Mode.

11.1 Sections Mandatory for a Genetic Informed Consent

In the following, modules being considered as an integral part of a Genetic IC are listed, and proposals for formulation of the respective sections are made, if adequate.

A genetic informed consent should include sections with respect to:
- Purpose of the study/research.

- Introduction to genetics.
- Expected benefits to the subjects and the community.
- Possible results.
- Potential risks.
- Storage of samples and derived data.
- Data protection and data security.
- Access to personal data.
- Risks if security measures are breached.
- Withdrawal.
- Independent review by Ethics Committees.
- Financial compensation.
- Different paragraphs for prespecified and unspecified mode.

11.1.1 Purpose of the Study

The specific purpose and objectives of the study should be clearly explained including both short-term objectives, i.e. evaluations, covered by the current informed consent, conducted immediately after the end of the study, and potential long-term applications, i.e. future possible planned evaluations that might be of interest.

A description of the disease(s) or clinical conditions of investigative interest during the current trial as well as those disorders of potential interest for study in the future should be provided.

Specify the genetic evaluations planned, but avoid a too itemized, too scientific description and wording. Explain, if ever possible, the goals of the intended analysis with plain words. The data subject must be able to comprehend it.

Proposal
Wording is dependent on study design and evaluations planned. A special proposal is therefore omitted, but the general considerations, outlined above, should be taken into account.

11.1.2 Introduction to Genetics

Briefly explain what is meant by genetics. Provide the basic ideas with understandable words, conceivable for all who have never heard of genetics before.

Proposal
It would be helpful to explain the benefits of genetic evaluations already done in the therapeutic area under consideration.

11.1.3 Expected Benefits to the Subject and the Community

Explain the benefits of the intended study for the individual participating patient and the community in general.

Proposal
Participating in this study will not result in any personal financial benefit, but we expect potential benefits for science and the community.
This study will give us more insight in the mechanism of [insert disease being considered in this study]. This might probably enable us to improve the treatment regimen and thus help other patients suffering from [insert disease being considered in this study] in the future. This study may allow scientists
- *to better understand why patients may respond differently to drugs received,*
- *to identify subjects who are not likely to benefit from a drug, prior to administration of that drug,*
- *to identify subjects who may experience side effects of a drug when this drug will be administered.*

11.1.4 Possible Results

Describe the possible outcomes of the intended genetic evaluations.

Proposal
Wording is dependent on the genetic evaluations planned. A special proposal is therefore omitted, but bear in mind that explanations must be understandable; use plain words.

11.1.5 Potential Risks

Explain both possible types of risks, physical as well as informational risks.

Proposal
The physical risks and discomfort of having blood taken from your vein include minor pain, bruising, fainting, or in rare cases, infection at the site where the blood was taken.
There may arise some concern that individual genetic information could be revealed to and might be misused by third parties. These concerns could include e.g. things like a possible denial of access to employment and insurances. [insert the sponsors' name] emphasizes that they will do everything to protect the subject's privacy, and ensures that all information derived from this study will never be inappropriately revealed to any third party. Taking however part in an anonymized genetic evaluation, there is no risk that genetic results could be revealed inappropriately. Genetic tests are carried out only after anonymization of samples and related clinical data, so that a trace back to your identity is no longer possible.

11.1.6 Storage of Samples and Derived Data

Describe how – storage devices, e.g. freezer, biobank, etc., where – location, e.g. company internal or external, and for what time – maximal timeframe that samples as well as derived data are stored for.

> **Proposal anonymized samples/data**
> Your consent participating in this study also includes that you agree with the storage of your [insert the biological material collected, e.g. blood, tissue, extracted DNA, etc.]. This material will be stored, as long as there is sufficient material to produce reliable results by applied scientific analysis (also for future research), but no longer than 10 years after the end of the respective study. The biological material will be processed and stored at [insert the institution/place where the material will be processed and stored]. Procedures are in place to protect your privacy. The only identifier of your DNA samples is a unique barcode.
> The same high protection level will be implemented for the genetic results derived from your samples. Access to genetic data is limited to authorized persons only. Moreover, anyone who has access to these results can only trace your identity to a coded identifier but not further. As your samples and data have passed an anonymization process, a trace back to your identity is impossible.
> All data collected on your behalf will be treated in compliance with [insert the respective legal framework, e.g. binding European directives and national/international laws].
>
> **Proposal de-identified samples/data**
> Your consent participating in this study also includes that you agree with the temporary storage of your [insert the biological material collected, e.g. blood, tissue, extracted DNA, etc.], if necessary. Your samples may be stored and used for genetic tests for up to 5 years after the end of the clinical trial. But during this time only tests for the purpose described above, also specified in the clinical trial protocol, can be done. As soon as the tests have been carried out, your samples will be destroyed.
> The biological material will be processed and stored at [insert the institution/place where the material will be processed and stored]. Procedures are in place to protect your privacy. The only identifier of your DNA samples is a unique barcode.
> The same high protection level will be implemented for the genetic results derived from your samples. Access to genetic data is limited to authorized persons only. Moreover, anyone who has access to these results can only trace your identity to a coded identifier but not further. Your doctor is the only person who actually knows your identity.
> All data collected on your behalf will be treated in compliance with [insert the respective legal framework, e.g. binding European directives and national/international laws].

11.1.7 Data Protection and Data Security

All intended uses of the genetic information and clinical information should be outlined and explained, i.e. it should be clearly specified in which way the results of the study will be handled.

This should include a section explaining that the results of the study may be sent to health authorities worldwide, or be used in study reports or in scientific presentations as well as in scientific publications.

The patient should be informed that a copy of results to be published may be obtained from the investigator on request, and that she/he will not be identified in any publication/presentation or report. It should be mentioned in addition that results of the study may also be used for future medical research.

Proposal
Genetic as well as clinical information may be transferred to
- *research partners, and/or business partners, and to*
- *regulatory authorities.*

Authorized persons from the sponsor, the regulatory agencies like the European Agency for the Evaluation of Medical Products (EMA), the U.S. Food and Drug Administration (FDA), or other governmental regulatory agencies, and/or the Ethics Committees may need to look at the medical records kept by your doctor to verify the information on the case report forms (source data verification), but they will not have access to your genetic results.
The results of the study may also be used in study reports, in scientific presentations or publications as well as for future medical research. In any case, your data are protected, you are not identified in any published collection of data and/or study results. Only de-identified data are used for those purposes throughout.

11.1.8 Access to Personal Data

Potential participants in a study should be advised of their rights and legal protections. This includes the right of being informed and the right of not being informed as well as possible consequences of getting individual study results. Explain that contracts with insurance companies might contain clauses that oblige the insurant to inform the insurer if a worsening of his state of health occurs. This may lead to a loss of the insurance if the worst comes to the worst.

> None love the bearer of bad news
> *Sophokles*

The results of any genetic analysis should be formulated within the limits of the objectives of the medical consultation, diagnosis or treatment for which consent was obtained. (cf. (43), section 6.2)

Proposal
You have the right to privacy, i.e. you may decide whether or not to be informed of information collected about your health.

If required, you will be informed of the results in so far as these correspond to the objectives of the consultation, of the diagnosis, or of the treatment, but you have the right to ask your doctor for more information in addition.

Your individual genetic results will not be given to your family, your general practitioner, your insurance company, and your employer or any other person or institution, unless this has been explicitly required by yourself or by law.

Being informed about the individual results may oblige you to inform your business partners like an insurance company due to paragraphs in existing or future insurance contracts. This might result in a cancellation of existing contracts or a refusal of future contracts.

11.1.9 Risks if Security Measures are Breached

Outline possible risks if an unexpected breach of the implemented security measures occurs. Explain how unlikely a breach will be and why. Describe your safeguards.

Proposal
In general, there will be no potential risks if security measures are breached.
The original key to trace back to the patient's identity (CDI) will be discarded during anonymization and replaced by a random identifier nCDI so that a trace back to the patient's identity will be no longer possible after anonymization.
The key to trace back to the patient's identity in case of de-identified data is held by the investigator. He is the only person who knows the relationship between the identifying key and the patient's identity.
In addition, the merging of both data sources for statistical evaluation purposes is a completely controlled and audit trailed process so that potential intruders are detected immediately and possible countermeasures can be initiated in due time.
All implemented security measures must successfully pass an itemized inspection process, being regularly executed. [insert the sponsors' name] emphasizes that all work is done in a controlled and validated environment, including software, hardware and the topology of the computing center involved.

11.1.10 Withdrawal – Options and Timelines

Emphasize the possibility for a patient to refuse his consent at any time, to withdraw it, and describe the consequences of such a withdrawal. Explain in particular that a withdrawal has no personal disadvantages.

Outline the possibility that a withdrawal may involve a request to destroy genetic material collected and to delete related genetic data created so far. Explain under which circumstances and up to what extent this can be realized and when.

Explain that a withdrawal from the genetic part of a clinical study does not necessarily imply a withdrawal from the clinical study itself. A withdrawal from the clinical part is a separate process.

On the other hand, a withdrawal from the clinical part of a study usually requires the deletion of respective clinical data collected so far, with the exception that regulatory guidelines and/or legal requirements prevent you to delete clinical information for a certain time. Genetic samples and derived genetic data become worthless if related clinical data are missing, that is why we can assume that a subject's withdrawal from the clinical part implicitly means also a withdrawal from the genetic part of the study. We therefore recommend you to kindly ask the respective patient, having withdrawn from the clinical part, whether this also means that she/he wants to withdraw from the genetic part, too. Remember that this does not belong to the contents of a genetic IC but rather to the contents of a related clinical IC. It is often overlooked, nevertheless important and thus worth mentioning.

Proposal for de-identified data
Participation in the study is entirely voluntary.
Taking part in this part of the study also includes that you may withdraw at any time without giving a reason.
There will be no change to any medical treatment you may be receiving if you should decide to withdraw from the study. You may in addition require your genetic material and derived genetic data collected so far to be destroyed. This will always be done in due time with the exception that there might be situations where regulatory guidelines and/or legal requirements do not allow to destroy samples and/or derived genetic data for a certain time period.
In any case, your data are highly protected; only the investigator can link the data to an individual patient and thus reveal your identity.

Proposal for anonymized data
Participation in the study is entirely voluntary.
Taking part in this part of the study also includes that you may withdraw at any time without giving a reason.
There will be no change to any medical treatment you may be receiving if you should decide to withdraw from the study. You may in addition require your genetic material and derived genetic data collected so far to be destroyed. This however is only possible as long as samples did not pass an anonymization process. Prior to anonymization no genetic data have been derived. After anonymization an identification of individual samples and/or data is no longer possible, and this implies that also a withdrawal can no longer be performed. This is by no means a disadvantage for you because anonymized samples/data are provided with the highest level of protection to privacy. A trace back to your identity is impossible.

11.1.11 Independent Review by Ethics Committees

Explain that the respective study has been reviewed and subsequently approved by Ethics Committees or Institutional Review Boards. Provide details which ECs and/or IRBs have been involved.

Outline the main tasks of ECs and/or IRBs with respect to the approval of the study considered.

Proposal
This study has been reviewed and approved by [insert the respective Ethics Committees and/or Institutional Review Boards]. This includes that the intended trial will be carried out within the ethical framework and that all your personal rights and welfare are protected.

11.1.12 Financial Compensation

Indicate any financial compensation for the participation. Outline who has the ownership of samples and scientific results. Make clear that there will be no further financial benefit if study results may be used in the development process of new drugs.

Proposal
No additional financial compensation will be paid for this part of the study. The results from this study might be valuable for commercial and/or intellectual property (patent) purposes. Any results obtained by the genetic analysis are exclusively owned by the sponsor.
You will not receive any compensation with respect to any commercial activities related to your genetic material including any interest in or share of any profits derived from the sale of any commercial test or drug made possible by your participation.
The sponsor is the sole owner of the research records, the research results, and the samples. However, as emphasized earlier, if you decide to withdraw your consent to this part of the study, your sample will be destroyed, if possible.

12 Selected Data Protection & Medical Sites

In the following, we provide selected links to data protection and medical sites. This should help the reader to easily locate the information needed. Laws, regulations, treaties as well as opinions and recommendations of legislative, regulatory, and scientific sites are accessible via the respective links.

Bear in mind that websites occasionally change their locators. This may be due to a revised technical layout and/or a complete redesign of the respective sites. We also observed that some sites reorganized completely the storage of their documents. Redirections to the new locations are sometimes provided, but this is by no means the standard.

In any case, all links provided below have been checked and work at time of publication of this book.

If you nevertheless observe a link that does not work in the course of time, we recommend to use the explanatory text of the websites as keywords to search the web for the respective site.

12.1 Germany

- Bundesministerium der Justiz – Gesetze im Internet
  http://bundesrecht.juris.de/index.html
- Der Bundesbeauftragte für den Datenschutz und die Informationsfreiheit
  http://www.bfdi.bund.de/Vorschaltseite_DE_node.html
  An English version of the site is also available via: http://www.bfdi.bund.de/EN/Home/homepage_node.html
  This site differs in content from the German page. Contents to be displayed on this site are considered to be of particular interest to international visitors.
- Datenschutzforum
  https://www.bfdi.bund.de/bfdi_forum/
- Virtuelles Datenschutzbüro
  http://www.datenschutz.de/
- Deutscher Ethikrat
  http://www.ethikrat.org/index
  An English version of this site is available via:
  http://www.ethikrat.org/publikationen/stellungnahmen
  The English versions of the publications are available via:
  http://www.ethikrat.org/publications/opinions/opinions?set_language=en
- Gesetze und Verordnungen des deutschen Bundesrechts im Internet
  http://www.buzer.de/index.htm
- Zentrale Kommission zur Wahrung ethischer Grundsätze in der Medizin und ihren Grenzgebieten, „Zentrale Ethikkommission"

http://www.zentrale-ethikkommission.de/
This site is available in German only.
- Unabhängiges Landeszentrum für Datenschutz Schleswig-Holstein
https://www.datenschutzzentrum.de/
This site is primarily available in German; only selected topics are presented in English.
- Bundesanzeiger – Bundesgesetzblatt
http://www.bgbl.de/index.php
This site is available in German only
- Deutsche Vereinigung für Datenschutz
https://www.datenschutzverein.de/
- BfArM: Bundesinstitut für Arzneimittel und Medizinprodukte
http://www.bfarm.de/EN/Home/home_node.html

12.2 Europe

- European Data Protection Supervisor (EDPS)
https://secure.edps.europa.eu/EDPSWEB/edps/lang/en/EDPS/Dataprotection
- European Union
    - EUR – Lex, Access to European Union law http://new.eur-lex.europa.eu/homepage.html?locale=en
    - Official Journal of the European Union http://eur-lex.europa.eu/JOIndex.do
    - European Union External Action http://eeas.europa.eu/eea/
- European Commission
    - European Commission: The European Union's Area of Freedom, Security, and Justice http://ec.europa.eu/justice/index_en.htm#newsroom-tab
    - European Commission: Justice/Data Protection http://ec.europa.eu/justice/data-protection/index_en.htm
    - European Commission: Justice/Data Protection/Documents http://ec.europa.eu/justice/data-protection/document/index_en.htm
    - European Commission: Justice/Data Protection/Article 29 Working Party http://ec.europa.eu/justice/data-protection/article-29/index_en.htm
    - European Commission: Justice/Data Protection/Article 29/Documentation
    The documents of the Article 29 Working Party: Opinions, Working Documents, Recommendations, Other documents, Annual Reports http://ec.europa.eu/justice/data-protection/article-29/documentation/index_en.htm
    Opinions can be accessed via:http://ec.europa.eu/justice/data-protection/article-29/documentation/opinion-recommendation/index_en.htm#h2-1
    - EU Commission – Documents Access http://ec.europa.eu/transparency/access_documents/index_en.htm

- EU Commission – Seventh Framework Programme (FP7) Getting Through Ethics Review: Ethics check list including informed consent aspects are available. http://cordis.europa.eu/fp7/ethics_en.html
    - EU Commission – Research & Innovation Horizon 2020 http://ec.europa.eu/research/horizon2020/index_en.cfm?pg=home#
    - CORDIS – Community Research and Development Information Service FP8: Towards the next Framework Programme http://cordis.europa.eu/fp7/ict/ssai/fp8preparations_en.html
- European Parliament
    - European Parliament: Charter of Fundamental Rights of the European Union http://www.europarl.europa.eu/comparl/libe/elsj/charter/art03/default_en.htm
    - European Parliament – Legislative Observatory Search http://www.europarl.europa.eu/oeil/search/search.do?lang=null
- Council of Europe
    - Council of Europe (COE) http://conventions.coe.int/
    - Complete list of the Council of Europe's treaties http://www.conventions.coe.int/Treaty/Commun/ListeTraites.asp?CM=8&CL=ENG
    - Search the COE documents http://www.coe.int/en/web/portal/google-search?q=R+%282002%29+9&sitesearch=coe.int&x=19&y=13
    - Council of Europe – Data Protection http://www.coe.int/t/dghl/standardsetting/DataProtection/default_en.asp
    - Access to Council documents: Public Register http://www.consilium.europa.eu/documents/access-to-council-documents-public-register?lang=en
    - European Court of Human Rights http://www.echr.coe.int/Pages/home.aspx?p=home&c
- European Medicines Agency
    - EMA European Medicines Agency (EMA was previously denoted EMEA) http://www.ema.europa.eu/ema/
    - EMA – Document Search http://www.ema.europa.eu/ema/index.jsp?curl=pages/document_library/landing/document_library_search.jsp&mid
    EMA – SOPs and Work Instructions
    Use Keyword Search and the document type filter "Work Instruction – Win"
    EMA – Documents with respect to Pharmacogenomics
    Use Keyword Search with "Pharmacogenomics" and the document types filter "All document types"
    EMA – GCP Documents
    Use Keyword Search with Keyword in Title "GCP" and the document types filter "All document types"
- Other
    - Epractice.eu: News – eGovernment, eInclusion, eHealth http://www.epractice.eu/en/news/

- EuroRec Institute http://www.eurorec.org/
- European Economic Area http://www.efta.int/eea
- European Society of Human Genetics – ESHG https://www.eshg.org/141.0.html
- EuroGentest – Harmonizing genetic testing across Europe http://www.eurogentest.org/
- Nuffield Council on Bioethics http://www.nuffieldbioethics.org/

12.3 US

- US Government Printing Office
  - US Government Printing Office http://www.gpo.gov/
  - Federal Register Main Page http://www.gpo.gov/fdsys/browse/collection.action?collectionCode=FR
  - Search GPO's Federal Digital System http://www.gpo.gov/fdsys/search/home.action
  - Electronic Code of Federal Regulations http://www.ecfr.gov/cgi-bin/text-idx?sid=f1a0e5fe33b3a84a2b7737cb2f267345&c=ecfr&tpl=/ecfrbrowse/Title45/45tab_02.tpl
- U.S. Department of Health and Human Services
  - U.S. Department of Health and Human Services http://www.hhs.gov/ocr/privacy/hipaa/administrative/privacyrule/index.html
  - U.S. Department of Health and Human Services – International, especially access the 2014 Edition of the International Compilation of Human Research Standards http://www.hhs.gov/ohrp/international/
  - U.S. Department of Health and Human Services, National Institutes of Health: HIPAA Privacy Rule http://privacyruleandresearch.nih.gov/
  - (HIPAA) Privacy Rule http://www.hhs.gov/ocr/privacy/
  - Institutional Review Boards (IRBs) -Site, Office for Human Research Protections (OHRP) http://www.hhs.gov/ohrp/assurances/irb/index.html
  - Office for Human Research Protections (OHRP), IRB Guidebook http://www.hhs.gov/ohrp/archive/irb/irb_guidebook.htm
  - Office for Human Research Protections (OHRP), Informed Consent Checklist http://www.hhs.gov/ohrp/policy/consentckls.html
  - U.S. Department of Health & Human Services/Regulations http://www.hhs.gov/regulations/
  - U.S. Department of Health & Human Services – Educational Material http://www.cms.gov/Regulations-and-Guidance/HIPAA-Administrative-Simplification/EducationMaterials/index.html?redirect=/EducationMaterials/02_HIPAAMaterials.asp#TopOfPage
- National Institute of General Medical Sciences

- National Institute of General Medical Sciences: First Community Consultation on the Responsible Collection and Use of Samples for Genetic Research http://www.nigms.nih.gov/News/Meetings/FirstCommunityConsultationResponsibleCollectionUseSamplesGeneticResearch.htm
    - National Institute of General Medical Sciences http://www.nigms.nih.gov/
- Export.gov
    - Export.gov: U.S.-EU & U.S.-Swiss Safe Harbor Frameworks http://export.gov/safeharbor/
    - Export.gov: Safe Harbor Documents http://export.gov/safeharbor/eg_main_018237.asp
    Especially, visit section II. EUROPEAN COMMISSION DOCUMENTS – July 28, 2000
    Letter from Commission Services transmitting the European Commission's Adequacy Finding
    European Commission's decision C(2000) 2441 finding the safe harbor to provide adequate protections
    Text on Non-Discrimination adopted by the Article 31 Committee on May 31, 2000
    Text on Non-Discrimination adopted by the Article 29 Working Party on February 3, 2000
    http://export.gov/safeharbor/eu/eg_main_018493.asp
    - Export.gov: European Union Safe Harbor Documents http://export.gov/safeharbor/eu/eg_main_018493.asp
- Food and Drug Administration
    - FDA: Genomics http://www.fda.gov/Drugs/ScienceResearch/ResearchAreas/Pharmacogenetics/default.htm
    - FDA: Code of Federal Regulations – Title 21 – Food and Drugs http://www.fda.gov/MedicalDevices/DeviceRegulationandGuidance/Databases/ucm135680.htm
    - FDA: Information Sheet Guidance for Institutional Review Boards (IRBs), Clinical Investigators, and Sponsors http://www.fda.gov/ScienceResearch/SpecialTopics/RunningClinicalTrials/GuidancesInformationSheetsandNotices/ucm113709.htm
    - FDA: A Guide to Informed Consent – Information Sheet Guidance for Institutional Review Boards and Clinical Investigators http://www.fda.gov/RegulatoryInformation/Guidances/ucm126431.htm
- Other
    - American Psychological Association: Frequently Asked Questions about Institutional Review Boards http://www.apa.org/about/gr/science/advocacy/2007/irbs.aspx
    - Genetics Home Reference – U.S. National Library of Medicine http://ghr.nlm.nih.gov/info=understandGenetics

- National Human Genome Research Institute http://www.genome.gov/
- Human Genome Project Information Archive 1990 – 2003 http://web.ornl.gov/sci/techresources/Human_Genome/posters/chromosome/index.shtml

12.4 Global Initiatives

- ICH Home
  - International Conference on Harmonisation of Technical Requirements for Registration of Pharmaceuticals for Human Use http://www.ich.org/
  - ICH Guidelines http://www.ich.org/products/guidelines.html
- GMP (Good Manufacturing Practices) Navigator (German) http://www.gmp-navigator.com/nav_link_navigator.html
- ECA – European Compliance Academy http://www.gmp-compliance.org/eca_index.html
- United Nations
  - United Nations, Human Rights http://www.ohchr.org/EN/Pages/WelcomePage.aspx
  - The Universal Declaration of Human Rights http://www.un.org/en/documents/udhr/index.shtml
- World Medical Association (WMA) – Declaration of Helsinki http://www.wma.net/en/20activities/10ethics/10helsinki/index.html
- CIOMS – Council for International Organizations of Medical Sciences http://www.cioms.ch/
- World Legal Information Institute http://www.worldlii.org/
- Electronic Privacy Information Center http://epic.org/
- The public voice http://thepublicvoice.org
- international database on Ethical, Legal and Social Issues in Human Genetics http://www.humgen.org/int/

The U.S. Department of Health & Human Services issues on its website HHS.gov the *International Compilation of Human Research Standards,* a listing of over 1000 laws, regulations, and guidelines on human subjects' protection in over 100 countries and from several international organizations. Many of the listings embed hyperlinks to the source documents. These laws, regulations, and guidelines are classified into seven categories:
1. General, i.e., applicable to most or all types of human subjects research.
2. Drugs and Devices.
3. Research Injury.

4. Privacy/Data Protection.
5. Human Biological Materials.
6. Genetic.
7. Embryos, Stem Cells, and Cloning.

(quotation from http://www.hhs.gov/ohrp/international/intlcompilation/intl-compilation.html)

The provided document is an excellent source, updated yearly.

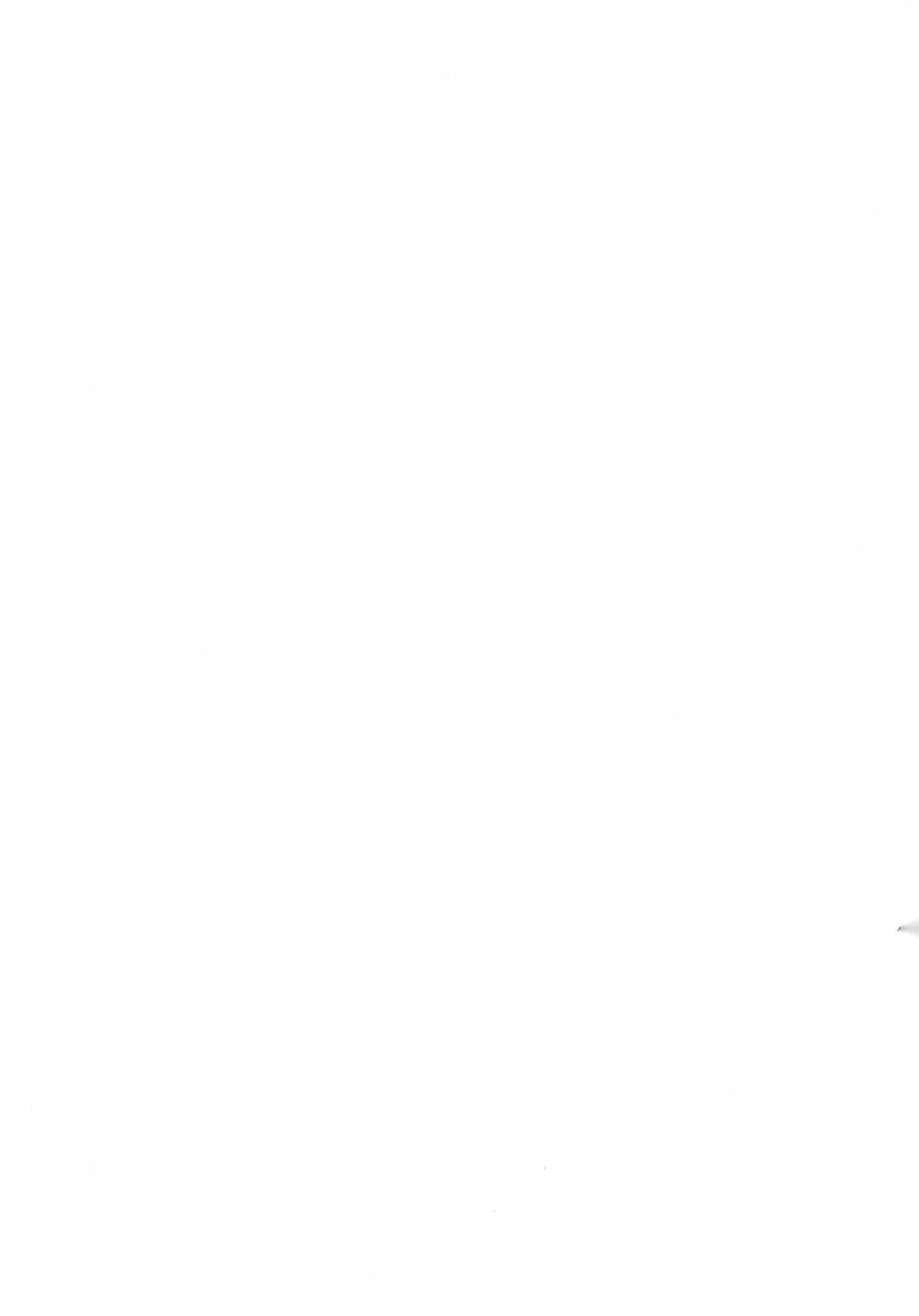

13 Impact of External Services on Data Protection

13.1 Introduction

Commissioned services like external sample management, with or without relabeling upon sample registration, DNA extraction, genetic testing, or statistical evaluations may have a high impact on an intended or already performed anonymization of clinical data and related genetic samples. Each external service used must therefore be critically analyzed in order to discover in which way and up to which extent the planned anonymization process or the existing anonymization is affected, respectively.

It is a general rule that a sample identifier the relation of which to GDI is known outside of the KPDB, must not be used as final identifier of samples, or as part of it, in the KPDB after anonymization.

Considering the whole sampling process as a four steps approach (Fig. 13.1):

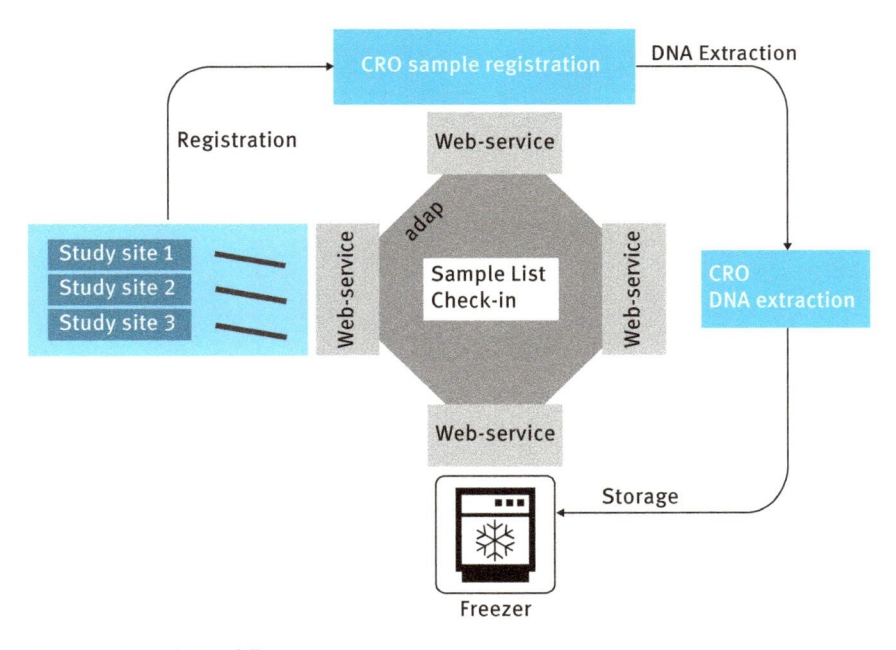

Fig. 13.1 Sample Workflow

- Collecting material at study sites and transferring it to the registration site,
- registration of material, performed by a registration CRO (regCRO) or by the staff of the sponsor,
- extraction of DNA, performed by an extraction CRO (exCRO) or by respective staff of the sponsor, and
- storing of DNA in a biobank,

enables us to easily discover potential weaknesses related to the applied labeling philosophy. Operations to be performed to guarantee a successful anonymization process later on, are more or less sophisticated and time-consuming. In the following we distinguish five possible scenarios:

Scenario 1: GDI label throughout, no label exchange.
Scenario 2: GDI label at study sites, label exchange upon registration, namely at CRO, but with remote access to sponsor system.
Scenario 3: GDI label at study sites, label exchange upon registration, namely locally at sponsor.
Scenario 4: GDI label at study sites, label exchange upon registration, namely at CRO with CRO system, new label CROSID from CRO.
Scenario 5: bSID label at study sites.

The respective tasks with respect to labeling and relabeling are summarized in table 13.1.

Tab. 13.1 Involving External Services – Label Exchange

	Study Site	Upon Registration	Upon DNA Extraction	Prior to Biobank Check-in
Scenario 1	GDI	GDI	GDI, RackID, r, c	GDI → nGDI RackID → nRackID
Scenario 2	GDI	GDI → nGDI	nGDI, RackID, r, c	no label exchange necessary
Scenario 3	GDI	GDI → nGDI	nGDI, RackID, r, c	
Scenario 4	GDI	GDI → CROSID	CROSID, RackID, r, c	CROSID → nGDI RackID → nRackID
Scenario 5	bSID	bSID	bSID, RackID, r, c	bSID → nGDI RackID → nRackID

Caption:

▮	GDI ↔ nGDI relationship is securely stored in the KPDB.
GDI	**G**enetic **D**ata **I**dentifier (contains PAT_NO)
nGDI	**n**ew **G**enetic **D**ata **I**dentifier (barcode)
CROSID	**S**ample **ID**entifier (CRO dependent labeling)
bSID	**b**arcoded **S**ample **ID**entifier (barcode)
RackID	DNA **R**ack **ID**entifier (barcode)
r	**r**ow position on rack (natural number)
c	**c**olumn position on rack (natural number)
nRackID	**n**ew DNA Rack **ID**entifier (barcode)
adap	**a**nonymization & **d**ata **p**rotection application.

The listed scenarios will be discussed in full detail below.

13.2 Scenario 1 – Using GDI Throughout

The first scenario assumes that the usual GDI label – PAT_NO based – will be attachedto the samples at study sites (Fig. 13.2).

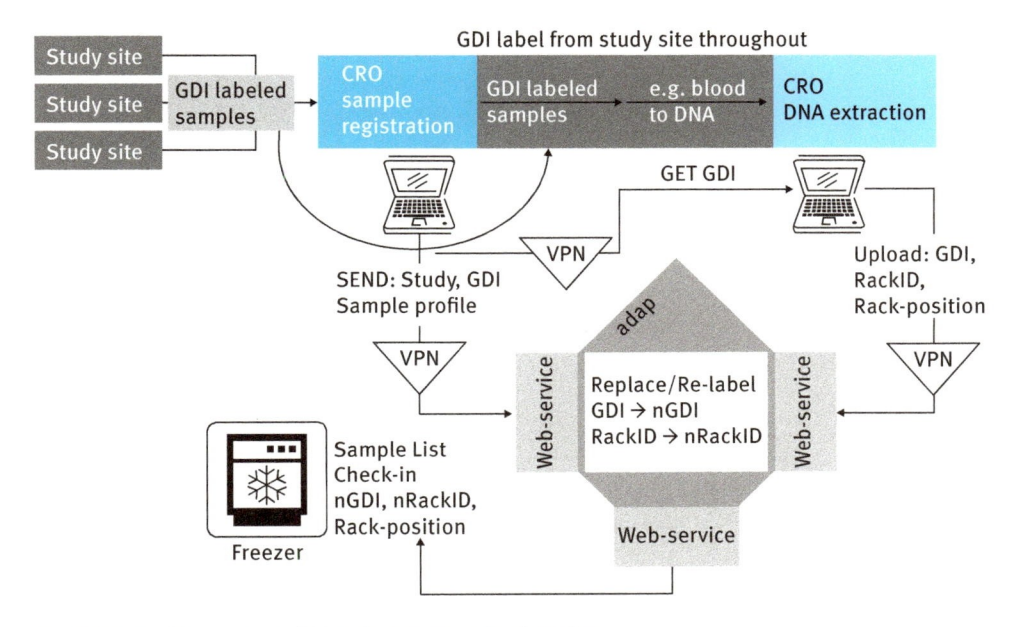

Fig. 13.2 Workflow – No Label Exchange upon Registration

The GDI, CDI relationship is recorded in the CRF/eCRF and stored in the clinical database. The GDI is still used as part of the identification of racks after DNA extraction. Prior to delivery of DNA racks to the biobank, RackID must be replaced by nRackID, and GDI must be replaced by nGDI in the keylist. You must check whether a replacement of the RackID is possible at all. It may be that the barcode is affixed. Bear in mind that pasting the new rackID over the old one is prohibited. Replacing the rack code is always a manual process whereas replacing GDI by nGDI is a KPDB service, performed electronically.

A sole replacement of GDI by nGDI is not sufficient, because the relationship RackID ↔ GDI is known by the extraction CRO, and a sole replacement of RackID is also not sufficient, because GDI is PAT_NO based and part of the DNA aliquots identification.

13.3 Scenario 2 – Replacing GDI by nGDI Upon Sample Registration, Performed by regCRO

The second scenario also assumes that the usual GDI label – PAT_NO based – will be attached to the samples at study sites (Fig. 13.3).

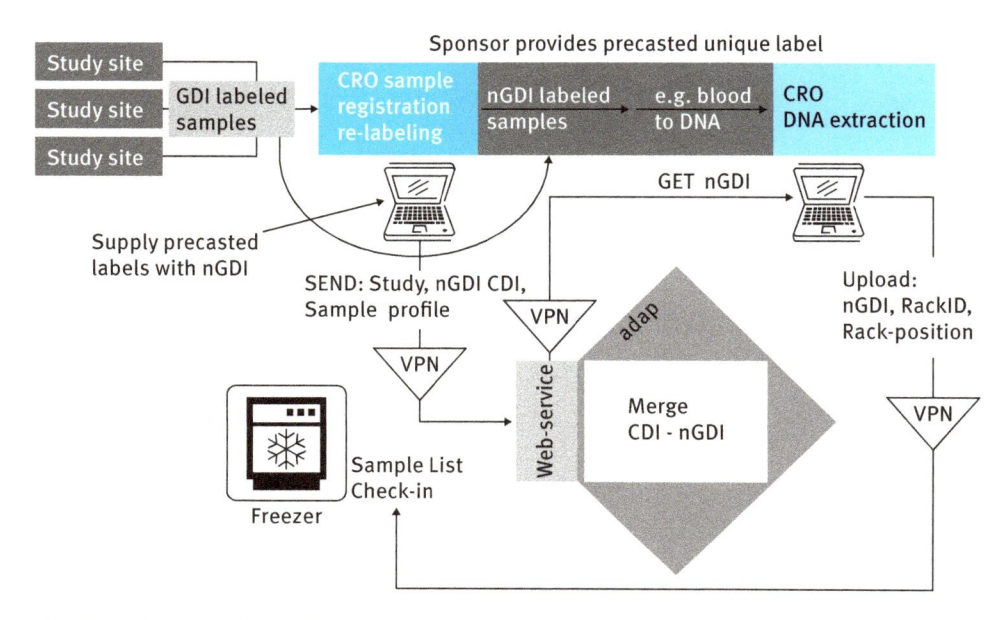

Fig. 13.3 Workflow – Label Exchange upon Registration

The GDI, CDI relationship is recorded in the CRF/eCRF and stored in the clinical database. Upon sample registration, the original GDI label is stripped off and replaced by a precasted nGDI label. Relabeling is performed by a registration CRO (regCRO) with remote access to the registration tool of the sponsor via a VPN line. The GDI, nGDI relationship is not recorded at the CRO but exclusively stored in the KPDB of the sponsor. It is recommended to additionally prohibit a handwritten recording of key relationships by contract. The nGDI is again used as part of the identification of racks after DNA extraction.

Prior to delivery of DNA racks to the biobank nothing is to relabel and/or to exchange.

A relabeling upon sample registration, replacing a PAT_NO based label by a nGDI barcode and securely storing the GDI ↔ nGDI relationship in the KPDB is sufficient for later anonymization.

13.4 Scenario 3 – Replacing GDI by nGDI Upon Sample Registration, Performed by Sponsor

Scenario 3 is essentially the same as scenario 2. The only difference is that relabeling is performed by the staff of the sponsor. We recommend to additionally implement a sample registration SOP that explicitly prohibits the handwritten recording of key relationships upon registration.

13.5 Scenario 4 – Sample Registration by CRO, Proprietary Labeling with CROSID

Scenario 4 again assumes that the usual GDI label – PAT_NO based – will be attached to the samples at study sites (Fig. 13.4). Relabeling of samples is performed by CRO employees using a proprietary registration system. The original GDI label is stripped off and replaced by a CRO proprietary CROSID label. The GDI, CROSID relationship and the sample profile information are sent to the anonymization system of the sponsor via a VPN line. Samples labeled with the CROSID are forwarded to the extraction CRO (exCRO) for DNA extraction. The CROSID is used furthermore as part of the identification of racks after DNA extraction. Prior to delivery of DNA racks to the biobank, RackID must be replaced by nRackID, and CROSID must be replaced by nGDI in the keylist. As before, you must check whether a replacement of the RackID is possible at all. It may be that the barcode is affixed.

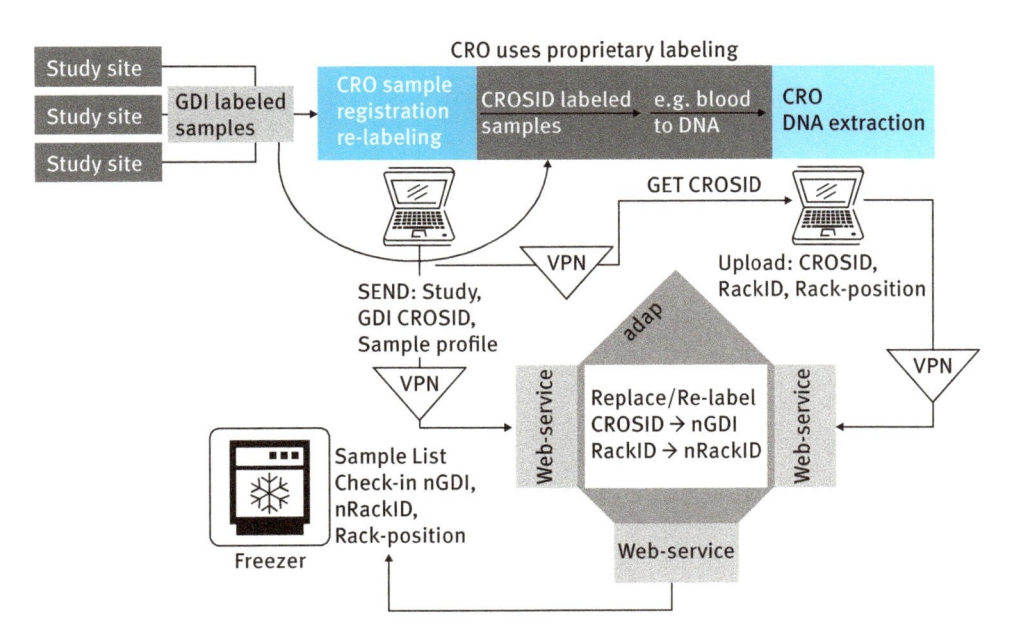

Fig. 13.4 Workflow – New CROSID Label upon Registration

A sole replacement of RackID is not sufficient, because the relationship CROSID ↔ GDI is known by the registration CRO.

A sole replacement of CROSID is also not sufficient, because the relationship CROSID ↔ RackID is known by the extraction CRO, and the CROSID ↔ GDI relationship is known by the registration CRO. A trace back to the patient's identity would thus be possible.

13.6 Scenario 5 – Barcoded Label bSID at Study Site

Scenario 5 assumes that labeling at study sites must be reorganized (Fig. 13.5).

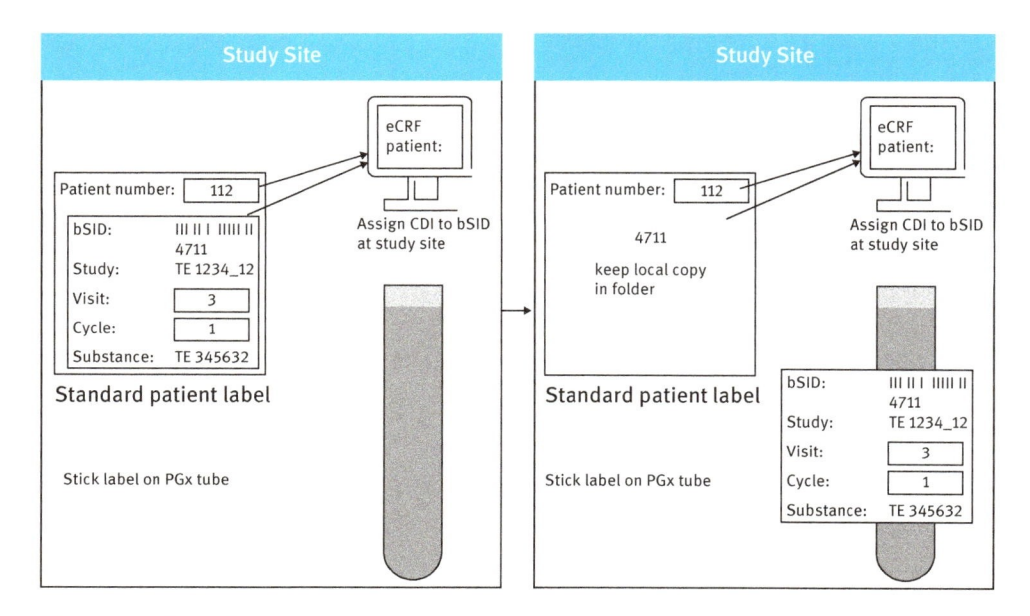

Fig. 13.5 bSID Labeling at Study Sites

The usual labeling of tubes with the patient number is replaced by new labels having already a precasted barcode bSID. This new label must be stuck on the collected tubes, and the PAT_NO, bSID relationship must be recorded in the CRF/eCRF (Fig. 13.6).

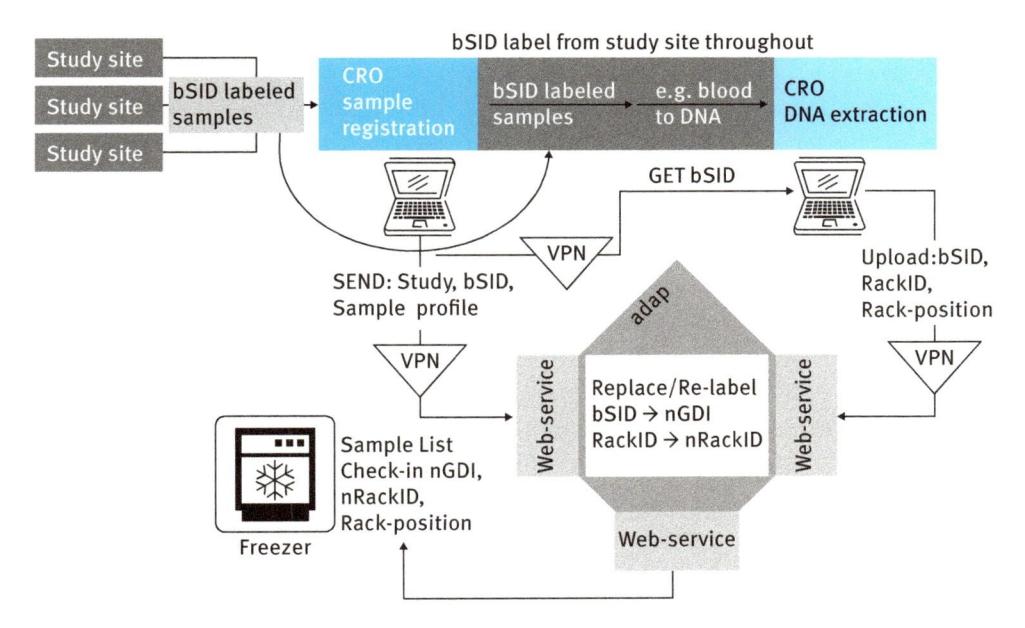

Fig. 13.6 Workflow – Barcoded bSID Label at Study Sites

bSID labeled samples are registered but not relabeled, and forwarded for DNA extraction to an extraction CRO. The bSID is used furthermore as part of the identification of racks after DNA extraction.

Prior to delivery of DNA racks to the biobank, RackID must be replaced by nRackID, and bSID must be replaced by nGDI in the keylist.

A sole replacement of RackID is not sufficient, because the relationship bSID ↔ PAT_NO is stored at the study site in the patient file and also in the clinical data base of the sponsor.

A sole replacement of bSID is also not sufficient, because the relationship bSID RackID is known by the extraction CRO, and the relationship bSID ↔ PAT_NO is stored at the study site in the patient file and also in the clinical data base of the sponsor. A trace back to the patient's identity would thus be possible.

13.7 Overall Summary

Scenarios 1, 4, 5 require a physical replacement of the rack code by a new rack code, and a respective replacement of GDI, CROSID, bSID by nGDI in the keylist.

Scenario 2, 3 require a relabeling of the collected blood tubes during registration but prior to forwarding the tubes to a DNA extraction CRO. A relabeling of racks and an additional exchange of keys in the keylist, prior to sending the DNA racks to the biobank for check-in process, is not necessary.

A delivery of barcoded labels to study sites would imply that the relation between CDI (includes PAT_NO) and the barcoded label is recorded via CRF or eCRF and thus stored in the de-identified clinical database. This again implies that during anonymization the barcode must be exchanged by a new one on all material, tubes, racks, etc. The replacement of this barcode must be done prior to check-in into a biobank, provided it is possible at all. The label exchange must be performed by a KPDB service and by no means by a biobank service, because the relationship old barcode – new barcode must not be stored in the biobank!

The delivery of barcoded labels to study sites would require local reorganizations and would mean no gain in data protection, but moreover supplementary work due to a relabeling of material prior to check-in into a biobank.

This implies that scenarios 1, 4, and 5 are not to be preferred. Scenarios 2 or 3, i.e. a relabeling upon sample registration is the best choice.

13.8 External Statistical Evaluation

An external statistical evaluation of anonymized clinical and related genetic data to be performed by a CRO can take place only after anonymization. The focus with respect to data protection therefore is on the avoidance of breaches of anonymization. It is important to make sure that the statistical evaluation of the de-identified counterpart of the data has not been performed by this CRO.

13.9 External Biobanking

The decision about external biobanking must be taken dependent on the case. It's closely related to your long-term strategy. A sporadic use of genetics does certainly not justify the installation of a private biobank. If genetics is an integral part of your research strategy, then external biobanking will probably prove as too cost intensive. Moreover the costs for transporting samples from an external biobank to the sponsor are not insignificant, and a repeated transport does not necessarily improve the quality of samples.

In any case, a cost benefit analysis should be performed prior to taking a long-term decision about biobanking.

14 Practical Approach to Clinical Trials with Supplementary Genetic Parts

14.1 Introduction

Initiating and performing clinical trials with supplementary genetic parts require an extensive work of planning and organizing. Dependent on the selected topology, distinct internal as well as external resources must be seamlessly assembled to successfully conduct the project. In any case, try to avoid a too scattered project topology, keep it simple. It's a general rule of thumb:

The more institutions are involved, the more complex the data protection layout will be.
The more external resources are involved, the more complex the data protection layout will be.

Boundary conditions and/or constraints to be taken into account are dependent on the actual data protection level of the data and/or samples collected. Prior to anonymization, processes are essentially governed by respective data protection laws, the clinical trial protocol, and the statistical analysis plan. After anonymization data protection laws only play a secondary role, because personal data have been converted to non-personal data, but in contrast prevention of privacy breaches, and Ethics Committee restrictions must be taken into account. A general prerequisite to prevent subjects from breaching anonymization is expressed by the following storage and access principles:
- De-identified and anonymized clinical data must be stored in separate databases.
- De-identified and anonymized genetic data must be stored in separate databases.
- Access to the same data sources with different protection masks is prohibited.

Access to clinical and related genetic data is either governed by the Clinical Trial Protocol or controlled by the genetic Review Board via the implemented request management (Fig. 14.1).

All external resources involved in a clinical project must be controlled by the sponsor as long as the protection level is "de-identified". Those itemized arrangements for inspection are in the first instance often required by law, secondly cost-intensive in general, and moreover time consuming.

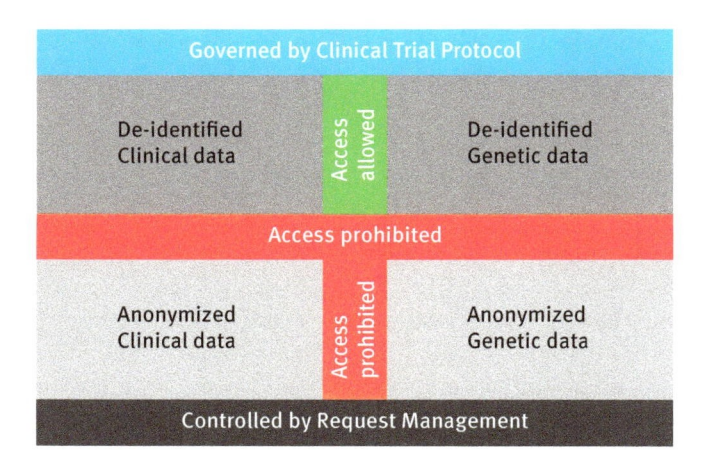

Fig. 14.1 Storage & Access Principles

Section 11 Collection, processing or use of personal data on behalf of others
(1) If other bodies collect, process or use personal data on behalf of the controller, the controller shall be responsible for compliance with the provisions of this Act and other data protection provisions. The rights referred to in Sections 6, 7 and 8 shall be asserted with regard to the controller.
(2) The processor shall be chosen carefully, with special attention to the suitability of the technical and organizational measures applied by the processor. The work to be carried out by the processor shall be specified in writing, including in particular the following:

1. the subject and duration of the work to be carried out,
2. the extent, type and purpose of the intended collection, processing or use of data, the type of data and category of data subjects,
3. the technical and organizational measures to be taken under Section 9,
4. the rectification, erasure and blocking of data,
5. the processor's obligations under subsection 4, in particular monitoring,
6. any right to issue subcontracts,
7. the controller's rights to monitor and the processor's corresponding obligations to accept and cooperate,
8. violations by the processor or its employees of provisions to protect personal data or of the terms specified by the controller which are subject to the obligation to notify,
9. the extent of the controller's authority to issue instructions to the processor,
10. the return of data storage media and the erasure of data recorded by the processor after the work has been carried out.

In case of public bodies, the work to be carried out may also be specified by the authority responsible for expert supervision. The controller shall verify compliance with the technical and organizational measures taken by the processor before data processing begins and regularly thereafter. The result shall be documented.
(3) The processor may collect, process or use the data only as instructed by the controller. If the processor believes that an instruction by the controller violates this Act or other data protection provisions, the processor shall inform the controller of this immediately.

(4) For the processor, other than Sections 5, 9, 43 (1) no. 2, Sections 10 and 11 (2) nos. 1 through 3 and (3), and Section 44, only the provisions on data protection monitoring or supervision shall apply, namely for
1. a) public bodies,
   b) private bodies, when the majority of shares or votes is publicly owned and the controller is a public body, Sections 18, 24 through 26 or the corresponding provisions of the data protection laws of the Länder,
2. other private bodies, where they collect, process or use personal data on behalf of others for commercial purposes as service providers, Sections 4f, 4g and 38.

(5) Subsections 1 through 4 shall apply accordingly if other bodies carry out the inspection or maintenance of automated procedures or data processing systems and the possibility of access to personal data during such inspection and maintenance cannot be ruled out.

Source: "Federal Data Protection Act (BDSG), In the version promulgated on 14 January 2003 (Federal Law Gazette I, p. 66), last amended by Article 1 of the Act of 14 August 2009 (Federal Law Gazette I, p. 2814)"

14.2 Overall Project Topology

The first and essential step when implementing a new clinical project with genetic addendum consists in the development of a rough summary of all services, mandatory for a successful realization. A stratification of services with respect to the categories "prior to" and "after anonymization" is meaningful, because laws and regulations to be applied are primarily dependent on these categories.

The diagram in Fig. 14.2 provides an example of how such an allocation of services could look like. In addition, services are grouped by the logical areas/tasks of the project considered.

In more detail, you must exactly determine:
- which services are to be included in the project,
and particularly:
- where these services are located and provided, either internally or externally.

This knowledge is important to plan and later initiate respective measures, required by regulations and laws.

Sample registration, DNA extraction, storage/biobank, conduct of genetic tests are services often provided internally, whereas sample collection is often commissioned to external logistic CROs. The commissioned collection can be arranged either with or without labeling service. These are two different approaches requiring also different data protection layouts. External labeling service has a high impact on data protection measures to be applied. We have analyzed the implications of this external service extensively in the preceding chapter.

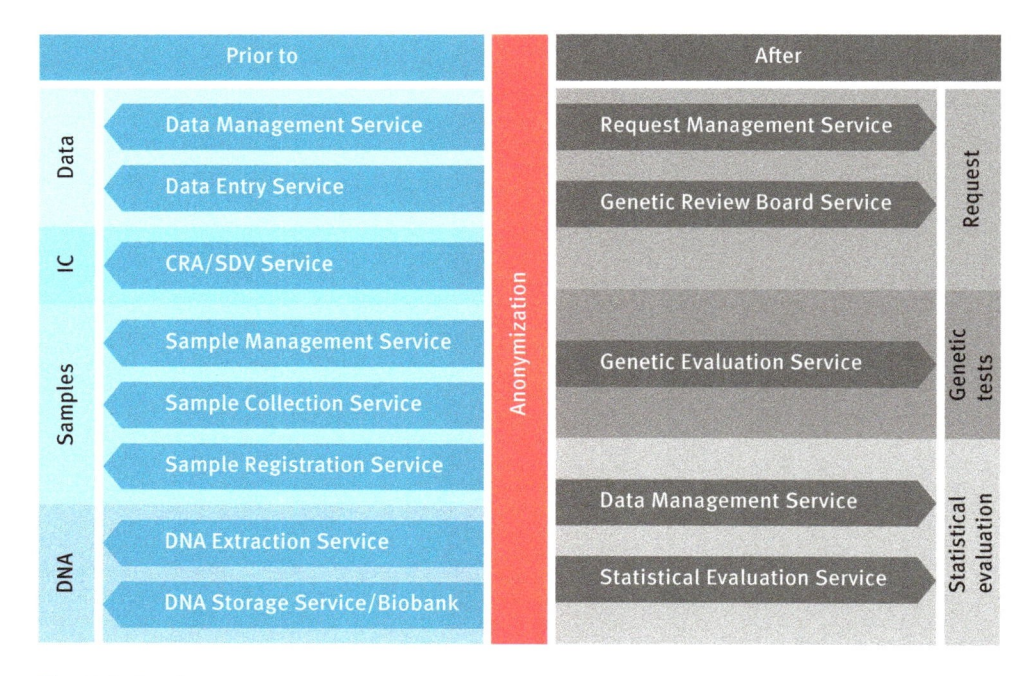

Fig. 14.2 Services

Statistical evaluation service is usually established as an internal service as well as Data Management service for preparing masking rules and data sets for anonymization. Request Management and Genetic Review Board (GRB) service are certainly internal services.

To support the reader to implement a structural approach to clinical trials with a supplementary genetic part we provide itemized checklists in the following, covering almost all organizational aspects like trial set-up, system topology, sample management, Informed Consent, Ethics Committee Restrictions, anonymization, and statistical evaluation.

14.3 Checklist – Trial Set-up

The *Trial Set-up Checklist* reminds the reader of the data protection issues that must be taken into consideration when planning national and/or multinational clinical trials having a genetic part, including countries with non-consolidated data protection laws.

Trial Set-up Checklist

1	What kind of clinical trial will be set up?		
	Screening Mode (genotyping)	YES ☐	NO ☐
	Prespecified Mode	YES ☐	NO ☐
	Unspecified Mode	YES ☐	NO ☐
	Prespecified Mode on the first stage and Unspecified Mode on the second stage	YES ☐	NO ☐
2	Do you plan the trial as multinational?	YES ☐	NO ☐
3	In case of a multinational trial: are only EU and/or EEA member states involved?	YES ☐	NO ☐
4	In case of an involvement of "third countries" (non EU or non EEA member states): did you already prepare contractual clauses?	YES ☐	NO ☐
5	Did you already involve your local data protection officer for Medicine?	YES ☐	NO ☐
6	Did you already check the respective genetic laws of countries where samples are planned to be collected?	YES ☐	NO ☐
7	Did you already check whether export of collected samples is allowed?	YES ☐	NO ☐
8	Is the data protection framework (distributed responsibility, access topology, etc.) already established?	YES ☐	NO ☐
9	Are you aware that de-identified and anonymized genetic data must be stored separately from each other?	YES ☐	NO ☐

Ad 6)
Countries having a specialized genetic law usually require also special procedures with respect to collection of genetic material and the subsequent statistical evaluation. Genetic labs must be authorized for the intended work in general.

Ad 7)
Some countries do not allow to export blood samples. DNA extraction and genetic evaluations must be performed locally. This issue must be taken into account, and respective measures must be initiated in due time.

Ad 9)
Temporary storage of genetic data in external systems, e.g. local LIMS of a CRO, should be planned very carefully. Data protection issues may arise if stored data must not be deleted later due to GLP requirements.

14.4 Checklist – System Topology

The *System Topology Checklist* supports the reader to examine whether all necessary system resources, hardware as well as software, are already available or available when actually needed.

	System Topology Checklist		
1	Are separate databases for de-identified and anonymized clinical data in place?	YES ☐	NO ☐
2	Are separate databases for de-identified and anonymized genetic data in place?	YES ☐	NO ☐
3	Is a validated (including 21 CFR Part 11) anonymization tool already available?	YES ☐	NO ☐
4	In case of internal sample management: Is a sample management tool available?	YES ☐	NO ☐
5	In case of internal sample registration: Is a sample registration software already implemented?	YES ☐	NO ☐
6	Is a special label printer available?	YES ☐	NO ☐
7	Is a lockable room for label printing already established?	YES ☐	NO ☐
8	How is DNA extraction planned?	internally ☐	externally ☐
9	Did you already think and decide about labeling of DNA aliquots?	YES ☐	NO ☐
10	How is DNA storage planned?	internally ☐	externally ☐
11	Did your company already install a validated software package for genetic analysis?	YES ☐	NO ☐
12	Did you already organize the access to all systems needed, taking into account that "anonymized" and "de-identified" groups must be separated from each other?	YES ☐	NO ☐

All questions should be answered with "YES", if adequate.

14.5 Checklist – Sample Management

The *Sample Management Checklist* is intended to clarify all questions in the context of sample management, sample collection, sample registration, and related topics. It is important to know whether single tasks are planned to be implemented as internal or external services. CRO involvement triggers audits with respect to quality and data protection aspects. In case of commissioned labeling and sample registration services we strongly recommend to carefully check whether experienced and qualified lab personnel is available at the CRO side, when needed. The respective employees must be able to master labeling, re-labeling, detach, and registration processes as a minimum. Permanent employees are to be preferred, compared to temporary workers. This decision should not be made subject to financial considerations. Quality is worth its price.

	Sample Management Checklist		
1	How is sample collection monitored?	internally ☐	externally ☐
2	How is sample registration performed?	internally ☐	externally ☐
3	In case of an external registration process: is registration performed with a CRO proprietary system (CRO proprietary labels) or via remote access to the sponsor's registration module (Sponsor labels)	CRO ☐	Sponsor ☐
4	In case of remote access: Did you already plan to provide the registration CRO with precasted nGDI labels?	YES ☐	NO ☐
5	In case of an external registration process: did you already determine how unplanned and additional samples will be dealt with?	YES ☐	NO ☐
6	Did you already implement a sample destruction process for samples having an unreadable labeling?	YES ☐	NO ☐
7	Where is DNA extraction performed?	internally ☐	externally ☐
8	Did you already implement an overall sample management – checking for completeness and correctness?	YES ☐	NO ☐
9	In case of CRO involvement: Are the commissioned tasks exclusively assigned to permanent employees?	YES ☐	NO ☐
10	In case of CRO involvement: Are quality audits already planned?	YES ☐	NO ☐
11	In case of CRO involvement: Are data protection audits already planned and/or organized?	YES ☐	NO ☐
12	In case of CRO involvement: Did you already check whether the respective CRO itself involves subcontractors?	YES ☐	NO ☐
13	In case of subcontractors involvement: Are the commissioned tasks exclusively assigned to permanent employees?	YES ☐	NO ☐

14	In case of subcontractors involvement: Are quality audits already planned?	YES ☐	NO ☐
15	In case of subcontractors involvement: Are data protection audits already planned and/or organized?	YES ☐	NO ☐
16	In case of CRO involvement: Did you plan temporary storage of material and data in such a way that GLP allows deletion at the CROs side after transferring data and collected material to the sponsor database and storage devices?	YES ☐	NO ☐
17	In case of CRO involvement: Did you already implement a sample destruction process (who and when) for samples having an unreadable labeling or samples having an unacceptable quality?	YES ☐	NO ☐

All questions should be answered with "YES", if adequate.

Ad 4)
Unplanned samples are samples taken at points in time not specified in the Clinical Trial Protocol.

Additional samples are samples additionally taken at planned points in time.

14.6 Checklist – ICs, Ethics Committees Restrictions

The *Informed Consent/EC Restrictions/Withdrawal Checklist* prompts you for topics needed in the context of IC management and for all possible restrictions Ethics Committees could impose.

Informed Consent/EC Restrictions/Withdrawal Checklist			
1	Is a separate genetic IC available?	YES ☐	NO ☐
2	Is a 100 % SDV planned for IC data?	YES ☐	NO ☐
3	Do you expect any objections to be raised by ECs with respect to therapeutic areas?	YES ☐	NO ☐
4	If "YES", did you already organize that genetic tests may be carried out only within the permitted range?	YES ☐	NO ☐
5	Do you expect any objections to be raised by ECs with respect to storage conditions?	YES ☐	NO ☐
6	If "YES", did you already establish a warning mechanism to guarantee that maximal allowed storage time is adhered?	YES ☐	NO ☐

7	Did you already implement a withdrawal process enter into force as from start of sample collection until anonymization?	YES ☐	NO ☐
8	Did you already implement a sample destruction process for samples related to a withdrawal or samples having exceeded the maximal storage time allowed?	YES ☐	NO ☐

14.7 Checklist – Anonymization

Prior to the start of the anonymization process all questions of the *Informed Consent/ EC Restrictions/Withdrawal Checklist* must have been answered with "YES". Remember that anonymization is an irreversible process, i.e. all necessary tasks like attaching of storage conditions and/or Ethics Committees restrictions to the data, solving of known withdrawal requests, and the subsequent destruction of samples concerned, must be carried out prior to anonymization.

	Anonymization Checklist		
1	Can you describe the anonymization process in detail so that regulatory authorities can comprehend it?	YES ☐	NO ☐
2	How will anonymization be guaranteed; e.g. how do you prevent subjects from matching anonymized and respective de-identified data? Are respective measures already in place?	YES ☐	NO ☐
3	Are you sure to have taken into account the privacy directives and, if available, genetic laws of all countries involved in your clinical study?	YES ☐	NO ☐
4	Did you check whether withdrawals have been completely solved?	YES ☐	NO ☐
5	Are masking rules already available?	YES ☐	NO ☐

All questions should be answered with "YES".

Ad 1)
You must be able to unambiguously describe the single steps of the anonymization process used. You must also prove that your process is compliant with 21 CFR Part 11, and you must be able to outline how anonymization is reached and how it is maintained.

14.8 Checklist – Statistical Evaluation

Prior to starting an evaluation of anonymized clinical and related genetic data some basic prerequisites must be met. The following *Evaluation Checklist* can be used to verify whether all necessary aspects have been taken into account.

	Evaluation Checklist		
1	Request Management established?	YES ☐	NO ☐
2	Genetic Review Board already in place?	YES ☐	NO ☐
3	Secure Evaluation Area (SEA) implemented?	YES ☐	NO ☐
4	Statistical group, exclusively responsible for analyzing anonymized data, already established?	YES ☐	NO ☐
5	Storage of results organized?	YES ☐	NO ☐
6	In case of external evaluation: Are the CRO, planned for evaluating the anonymized data, and the CRO which did already evaluate the de-identified clinical data different?	YES ☐	NO ☐
7	In case of an internal evaluation either in the operative unit responsible for the trial or in another operative unit of your company, etc.: Are the group, planned for evaluating the anonymized data, and the group which did already evaluate the de-identified data different?	YES ☐	NO ☐

All questions should be answered with "YES"

Ad 6) and Ad 7)
Clinical and related genetic data did pass the anonymization process, i.e. they are no longer personal data and thus not subject to data protection requirements, provided that anonymization will not be breached. To prevent a breach of anonymization by simply matching anonymized data with their de-identified counterparts it is absolutely necessary that the correct access rules have been implemented.

Appendix

Appendix 1	Data Protection in the European Union
Appendix 2	Data Types
Appendix 3	Protection Masks
Appendix 4	Informed Consent (IC)
Appendix 5	Security

15 Appendix 1: Data Protection in the European Union

15.1 Council of Europe (COE)

The Council of Europe was founded in the late 1940s as an intra-European human rights organization. The COE documents are complementing the privacy protection provision of the ECHR (*European Convention on Human Rights*) and lay down modern data protection standards.

15.2 EU Privacy Directive – Definitions

In its article 2 – definitions – the EU privacy Directive defines basic terms used in the context of data protection.

(a) **'personal data'** shall mean any information relating to an identified or identifiable natural person ('data subject'); an identifiable person is one who can be identified, directly or indirectly, in particular by reference to an identification number or to one or more factors specific to his physical, physiological, mental, economic, cultural or social identity;

(b) **'processing of personal data'** ('processing') shall mean any operation or set of operations which is performed upon personal data, whether or not by automatic means, such as collection, recording, organization, storage, adaptation or alteration, retrieval, consultation, use, disclosure by transmission, dissemination or otherwise making available, alignment or combination, blocking, erasure or destruction;

(c) **'personal data filing system'** ('filing system') shall mean any structured set of personal data which are accessible according to specific criteria, whether centralized, decentralized or dispersed on a functional or geographical basis;

(d) **'controller'** shall mean the natural or legal person, public authority, agency or any other body which alone or jointly with others determines the purposes and means of the processing of personal data; where the purposes and means of processing are determined by national or Community laws or regulations, the controller or the specific criteria for his nomination may be designated by national or Community law;

(e) **'processor'** shall mean a natural or legal person, public authority, agency or any other body which processes personal data on behalf of the controller;

(f) **'third party'** shall mean any natural or legal person, public authority, agency or any other body other than the data subject, the controller, the processor and the persons who, under the direct authority of the controller or the processor, are authorized to process the data;

(g) **'recipient'** shall mean a natural or legal person, public authority, agency or any other body to whom data are disclosed, whether a third party or not; however, authorities which may receive data in the framework of a particular inquiry shall not be regarded as recipients;

(h) **'the data subject's consent'** shall mean any freely given specific and informed indication of his wishes by which the data subject signifies his agreement to personal data relating to him being processed

15.3 Tasks of the Article 29 Data Protection Working Party

Articles 29 and 30 of Directive 95/46/EC, Official Journal L 281, 23/11/1995 p. 0031 – 0050

Article 29
Working Party on the Protection of Individuals with regard to the Processing of Personal Data
1. A Working Party on the Protection of Individuals with regard to the Processing of Personal Data, hereinafter referred to as 'the Working Party', is hereby set up. It shall have advisory status and act independently.
2. The Working Party shall be composed of a representative of the supervisory authority or authorities designated by each Member State and of a representative of the authority or authorities established for the Community institutions and bodies, and of a representative of the Commission.
   Each member of the Working Party shall be designated by the institution, authority or authorities which he represents. Where a Member State has designated more than one supervisory authority, they shall nominate a joint representative. The same shall apply to the authorities established for Community institutions and bodies.
3. The Working Party shall take decisions by a simple majority of the representatives of the supervisory authorities
4. The Working Party shall elect its chairman. The chairman's term of office shall be two years. His appointment shall be renewable
5. The Working Party's secretariat shall be provided by the Commission.
6. The Working Party shall adopt its own rules of procedure.
7. The Working Party shall consider items placed on its agenda by its chairman, either on his own initiative or at the request of a representative of the supervisory authorities or at the Commission's request.

Article 30
1. The Working Party shall:
   (a) examine any question covering the application of the national measures adopted under this Directive in order to contribute to the uniform application of such measures;
   (b) give the Commission an opinion on the level of protection in the Community and in third countries;
   (c) advise the Commission on any proposed amendment of this Directive, on any additional or specific measures to safeguard the rights and freedoms of natural persons with regard to the processing of personal data and on any other proposed Community measures affecting such rights and freedoms;
   (d) give an opinion on codes of conduct drawn up at Community level.
2. If the Working Party finds that divergences likely to affect the equivalence of protection for persons with regard to the processing of personal data in the Community are arising between the laws or practices of Member States, it shall inform the Commission accordingly.
3. The Working Party may, on its own initiative, make recommendations on all matters relating to the protection of persons with regard to the processing of personal data in the Community.

4. The Working Party's opinions and recommendations shall be forwarded to the Commission and to the committee referred to in Article 31.
5. The Commission shall inform the Working Party of the action it has taken in response to its opinions and recommendations. It shall do so in a report which shall also be forwarded to the European Parliament and the Council. The report shall be made public.
6. The Working Party shall draw up an annual report on the situation regarding the protection of natural persons with regard to the processing of personal data in the Community and in third countries, which it shall transmit to the Commission, the European Parliament and the Council. The report shall be made public.

Article 14 of Directive 97/66/EC of the European Parliament and of the Council of 15 December 1997 concerning the processing of personal data and the protection of privacy in the telecommunications sector, Official Journal L 024 , 30/01/1998 p. 0001 – 0008

Article 14
Extension of the scope of application of certain provisions of Directive 95/46/EC

3. The Working Party on the Protection of Individuals with regard to the Processing of Personal Data established according to Article 29 of Directive 95/46/EC shall carry out the tasks laid down in Article 30 of the above mentioned Directive also with regard to the protection of fundamental rights and freedoms and of legitimate interests in the telecommunications sector, which is the subject of this Directive.

As laid down in DIRECTIVE 2002/58/EC of 12 July 2002, concerning the processing of personal data and the protection of privacy in the electronic communications sector, denoted as Directive on privacy and electronic communications, usually briefly referred to as the **ePrivacy Directive**, cf. p.37 (4)

Directive 97/66/EC of the European Parliament and of the Council of 15 December 1997 concerning the processing of personal data and the protection of privacy in the telecommunications sector (5) translated the principles set out in Directive 95/46/EC into specific rules for the telecommunications sector. Directive 97/66/EC has to be adapted to developments in the markets and technologies for electronic communications services in order to provide an equal level of protection of personal data and privacy for users of publicly available electronic communications services, regardless of the technologies used. That Directive should therefore be repealed and replaced by this Directive.

16 Appendix 2: Data Types

16.1 EU Privacy Directive (October 24, 1995)

(a) **'personal data'** shall mean **any information relating to an identified** or **identifiable natural person ('data subject')**; an identifiable person is one who can be identified, **directly** or **indirectly**, in particular by reference to an identification number or to one or more factors specific to his physical, physiological, mental, economic, cultural or social identity;

16.2 Council of Europe (COE) Definition of Data Types

(cf. (43), Appendix to Recommendation No. R (97) 5)

1. Definitions

For the purposes of this recommendation:
- the expression "personal data" covers any information relating to an identified or identifiable individual. An individual shall not be regarded as "identifiable" if identification requires an unreasonable amount of time and manpower. In cases where the individual is not identifiable, the data are referred to as anonymous;
- the expression "medical data" refers to all personal data concerning the health of an individual. It refers also to data which have a clear and close link with health as well as to genetic data;
- the expression "genetic data" refers to all data, of whatever type, concerning the hereditary characteristics of an individual or concerning the pattern of inheritance of such characteristics within a related group of individuals.

It also refers to all data on the carrying of any genetic information (genes) in an individual or genetic line relating to any aspect of health or disease, whether present as identifiable characteristics or not.

The genetic line is the line constituted by genetic similarities resulting from procreation and shared by two or more individuals.

3.2. Medical data may only be collected and processed if in accordance with appropriate safeguards which must be provided by domestic law.

Comment:
Even though its title refers to "medical" data, the Recommendation given in Article 1 emphasizes clearly that it covers health data broadly:

The expression **"medical data"** refers to **all personal data concerning the health** of an individual. It also refers to data, which have a clear and close link with health **as well as to genetic data**.

The Recommendation's concerns are to protect personally identifiable data, but it notes (Article 1): "An individual shall not be regarded as 'identifiable' if identification requires an unreasonable amount of time and manpower." The respective data are considered to be anonymous.

Genetic data

4.7. Genetic data collected and processed for preventive treatment, diagnosis or treatment of the data subject or for scientific research should only be used for these purposes or to allow the data subject to take a free and informed decision on these matters.

4.8. Processing of genetic data for the purpose of a judicial procedure or a criminal investigation should be the subject of a specific law offering appropriate safeguards
The data should only be used to establish whether there is a genetic link in the framework of adducing evidence, to prevent a real danger or to suppress a specific criminal offence. In no case should they be used to determine other characteristics which may be linked genetically.

4.9. For purposes other than those provided for in Principles 4.7 and 4.8, the collection and processing of genetic data should, in principle, only be permitted for health reasons and in particular to avoid any serious prejudice to the health of the data subject or third parties. However, the collection and processing of genetic data in order to predict illness may be allowed for in cases of overriding interest and subject to appropriate safeguards defined by law.

Some more explanations are given in (44), in the Explanatory Memorandum to Recommendation No. R (97) 5.

Genetic data

89. In spite of the specific nature of genetic data (see paragraphs 41-58 above), the drafters of the recommendation considered that the conditions for their collection and processing should be the same as those for the collection and processing of medical data, set out in Principle 4.3.

90. In this connection, the drafters of the recommendation were aware that the collection and processing of genetic data may be necessary in the interests not only of the protection of public health, but also the promotion of public health, since genetic analyses might reveal health risks for future generations. They were aware, however, that this possibility should not lead to a proliferation of genetic databanks, or an abuse of genetic data.

91. Principle 4.1, inspired by Article 5 of the convention, implies that genetic data may be processed only for purposes compatible with the purposes for which they were collected, and on the same conditions. The drafters of the recommendation did not include a requirement that genetic data should not be used for artificial modifications of the genetic heritage of data subjects, cloning or the selection of individuals, since such requirement would seem to be outside the scope of the recommendation, and is, in any case, covered by the principle of compatible purposes.

92. Genetic data collected and processed for diagnosis or medical or preventive treatment or for scientific research purposes, should only be used, in the first instance, for these specific purposes or to enable the data subject to take a decision whether or not to undergo treatment; the same principle applies when the data were collected with a view to procreation. Principle 4.7 is a logical consequence of the general principle of purpose specification; to use or reuse such data for other purposes should not be allowed. Principle 4.7 also applies when genetic analysis is carried out to establish whether a person can procreate without risk to the health of his/her future children. In this respect, Principle 4.7 does not aim at establishing an ethical norm on whether or not procreation should be preceded by genetic analysis; the principle merely requires that if genetic data are collected for that purpose in accordance with domestic law or the existing ethical standards, they may be used only to facilitate the data subject's decision.

93. In defining Principle 4.7 the drafters of the recommendation paid special attention to the use of genetic data for scientific research; in this context they confirmed that such research would be ruled by Chapter 12 "Scientific research". It was agreed that secondary use for scientific research of genetic data which had been collected for other purposes would not be incompatible with these initial purposes, as long as the conditions in Chapter 12 were respected, in particular Principle 12.2 (see paragraphs 200-209 hereafter) and Principle 12.3 (paragraph 209).

94. Principle 4.7, which applies to scientific research in general, is followed by two principles aimed more specifically at situations where genetic analysis may be carried out with a specific aim.

95. Although the analysis of deoxyribonucleic acid (DNA) within the framework of criminal justice is regulated in Recommendation No. R (92) 1, adopted by the Committee of Ministers on 10 February 1992, the drafters of the recommendation considered it useful to include in this recommendation a provision on the protection of genetic data processed for the purpose of criminal investigations, which also covers analysis of such data for the requirements of judicial procedures.

96. The expression "judicial procedure" is not used in the same way in member states. The drafters of the recommendation wished Principle 4.8 to apply to any procedure before the courts, whether initiated under civil or criminal law, where the judicial proceedings may have recourse to genetic analysis of one or more persons.

97. Consequently, Principle 4.8 requires a specific law for the processing of genetic data for judicial procedures and criminal investigations. By "specific law" is understood either a specific provision of the data protection act, or a specific provision in penal law, as long as they refer to the use of genetic data for the purpose of criminal investigations. This requirement is a logical consequence of Article 6 of the convention which imposes appropriate safeguards in domestic law for the processing of any sensitive data. The principle of compatibility of purposes also applies here: data collected and processed in the framework of judicial procedures and criminal investigations shall be used only for the original purposes and not for other purposes, in particular not to determine other characteristics of the data subject (see paragraph 78 above).

98. The second paragraph of Principle 4.8 is intended to define these purposes. Genetic data processed for the needs of a judicial procedure, for example a paternity suit, should be used only to establish whether or not there is a genetic link between the child and the alleged father. In the same way, in a criminal investigation genetic data should be used only in order to prevent a real danger or suppress a criminal offence.

99. It was considered that the proof of guilt or innocence, even on the basis of evidence supplied by genetic analyses, would be beyond the scope of this recommendation.

100. Principle 4.9 aims at regulating the use of genetic data for purposes other than diagnosis, therapeutic or preventive treatment, scientific research or criminal investigations. This use can only be allowed in principle for health reasons and to avoid every serious risk for the health of the data subject or for a third person. However, in the case of the collection and processing of genetic data in order to predict illness, the recommendation requires the existence of an overriding interest and appropriate safeguards provided for by law in view of the various risks inherent in the collection and processing of genetic data, in particular the risk of discrimination (as far as reference to law is concerned, in view of the case-law of the organs of the European Convention on Human Rights, see paragraph 75 of the present explanatory memorandum).
101. It should be recalled that the conditions for lawfulness laid down in Principle 4.3 also apply to the collection and processing of genetic data.
102. Principle 4.10 adds a supplementary condition for genetic data to be collected and processed: the purpose of collection and processing must be health protection and in particular the prevention of any serious harm to the data subject or a third person.
103. The drafters of the recommendation emphasised that a candidate for employment, an insurance contract or other services or activities should not be forced to undergo a genetic analysis, by making the employment or the insurance dependent on such analysis, unless such dependence is explicitly provided for by law and the analysis is necessary for the protection of the data subject or a third party (for example work with dangerous substances).
104. Principle 4.9 is even more specific with regard to the collection and processing of genetic data with a view to predicting illness. Such data may be collected and processed if the interest in doing so overrides the data subject's interest in not having his/her genetic data collected and processed (for example a collective interest) and if domestic law has provided appropriate safeguards. It was understood that such overriding interest should be in accordance with the related criteria set out in Principle 4.3.

16.3 Federal Data Protection Act (GER) as of 1. Jan. 2003

Section 3, Further definitions
(1) "Personal data" means any information concerning the personal or material circumstances of an **identified** or **identifiable** individual (the data subject).

17 Appendix 3: Protection Masks

17.1 EMA definition of anonymous sample/data

(cf. (7) EMEA, understanding the terminology used in pharmacogenetics)

Anonymous samples and results
Your sample on which to carry pharmacogenetic testing, is taken for research purposes and there is no link with your identity: samples and data are defined as '**anonymous**'. This type of collecting and coding of samples is usually only used for general medical research.

This way of handling samples and genetic data only allows for the link between the genetic results and the clinical record but not to your identity. It gives the highest level of additional privacy protection, but also implies that you might not be able to withdraw your sample from further analyses or receive your individual results from the study.

This also has an additional consequence – regulatory authorities in charge of Good Clinical Practices in clinical trials will have no opportunity to check how accurate and reliable the pharmacogenetic results are, as there may be times when they need to check and link a clinical response to a particular participant and his or her genetic profile.

Comment: This definition differs from the COE Recommendation No. R (97) 5 (cf. (43)).

17.2 Germany

17.2.1 Anonymization (Rendering anonymous) and De-Identification (Aliasing)

(cf. Federal Data Protection Act (as of 1 January 2003))

In section 3 Further Definitions, 6, 6a the **anonymization (Rendering anonymous)** and **de-identification (Aliasing)** process have been defined.

- (6) "**Rendering anonymous**" means the modification of personal data so that the information concerning personal or material circumstances can no longer or only with a disproportionate amount of time, expense and labour be attributed to an identified or identifiable individual.
- (6a) "**Aliasing**" means replacing a person's name and other identifying characteristics with a label, in order to preclude identification of the data subject or to render such identification substantially difficult.

17.2.2 Further Recommendations, not yet Regulations

62. Konferenz der Datenschutzbeauftragten des Bundes und der Länder (Münster, 24.-26. Oktober 2001)
(Auszug aus: Anlage zur Entschließung gesetzliche Regelung von genetischen Untersuchungen; Vorschläge zur Sicherung der Selbstbestimmung bei genetischen Untersuchungen, cf. (35))

Begriffe

1. Genetische Untersuchungen: Untersuchungen auf Chromosomen-, Genprodukt- oder molekularer DNS/RNS-Ebene, die darauf abzielen, Informationen über das Erbgut zu erhalten
8. Genetische Daten: im Zusammenhang mit genetischen Untersuchungen erlangte Informationen über eine Person;

Datensicherheit
(1) Proben und genetische Daten sind vor dem Zugriff unbefugter Dritter wirksam zu schützen. Dies gilt auch in Bezug auf Mitarbeiterinnen und Mitarbeiter der untersuchenden und datenverarbeitenden Stelle, die an der genetischen Untersuchung, Aufklärung und Beratung nicht beteiligt sind oder waren.
(2) Genetische Daten sind von anderen Datenarten gesondert zu speichern.
(3) Im Übrigen gilt hinsichtlich der genetischen Daten die Bestimmung des Bundesdatenschutzgesetzes über die technischen und organisatorischen Maßnahmen der Datensicherheit in der jeweils geltenden Fassung

17.3 Spain

ORGANIC LAW 15/1999 of 13 December on the Protection of Personal Data (published in the Boletín Oficial del Estado, no. 14, of 14 December 1999), at art. 3(f): 'Procedimiento de disociación' (cf. (41)).

In Spain the process of **anonymization** is defined under the **data protection law** in the following terms:

> "Dissociation procedure: any processing of personal data carried out in such a way that the information obtained cannot be associated with an identified or identifiable person."

17.4 US

17.4.1 William W. Lowrance, Privacy and Health Research

A Report to the U.S. Secretary of Health and Human Services, May 1997, (cf. (42))

> **ANONYMIZED DATA**
> Much very useful health research is performed on completely anonymized data. If for a particular research project there are no compelling reasons for retaining at least potential identifiability, anonymized data should be used. Though this injunction might sound unnecessary, it is stated here because often, data with identifiers are used just because they happen already to be on hand in identified form.
> Data may be non-identifiable if any of the following tactics have been employed:
> - Identifiers simply have never been collected.
> - Identifiers have been removed ("stripped") effectively.
> - Data have been aggregated – that is, within each data subelement the data have been averaged or grouped into ranges, and only the averages or ranges reported, not revealing the identity of the data-subjects.
> - Data have been "micro-aggregated," with small randomly assembled clusters of cases averaged, in effect generating a set of pseudocases that represent the real population.
>
> The test of whether data actually are non-identifiable is whether a person without prior knowledge of the data or their collection can, from the data and any other available information (such as postal-code charts, or a casually held key to a code, or a list of the people recruited to the study), deduce the personal identity of data-subjects.
>
> Samples are anonymous if and only if it is impossible under any circumstances to identify the individual source. At present, in settings such as those involving large population groups, it may be possible to ensure anonymity while retaining some information about the individual source, such as ethnic origin, sex, age cohort, or limited clinical data, with the sample. In other settings, such as DNA samples obtained from a small group of individuals at risk for a specific disorder, retention of additional information may compromise anonymity. Samples are not anonymous if it is possible for any person to link the sample with its source. Even if the researcher cannot identify the source of the tissue, the samples are not anonymous if some other individual or institution has the ability.
>
> U.S. agencies, such as the National Heart, Lung, and Blood Institute (NHLBI), emphasize that the first step in protecting personally identifiable data is simply to hold the identifiers close to the point of collection.
>
> Before transferring data to other researchers, then, the data should be stripped of identifiers and either keycoded or anonymized. When the Institute sends data to pharmaceutical companies from clinical trials on an investigational new drug, it strips off not only the patient and physician name but location, birthdate, and other data that could point back to the data-subject. It takes similar care when it correlates data from several sources, as when it links heart disease data with socioeconomic data.

17.4.2 HIPAA Privacy Rules

(HIPAA – Health Insurance Portability and Accountability Act, Standards for Privacy of Individually Identifiable Health Information, 45 CFR Parts 160 and 164, (12))

2. Limited Data Sets
From the de-identification safe harbour list of identifiers, we proposed the following as direct identifiers that would have to be removed from any limited data set:
name, street address, telephone and fax numbers, e-mail address, social security number, certificate/license number, vehicle identifiers and serial numbers, URLs and IP addresses, and full face photos and any other comparable images. The proposed limited data set could include the following identifiable information: admission, discharge, and service dates; date of death; age (including age 90 or over); and five-digit zip code.
The Department solicited comment on whether one or more other geographic units smaller than State, such as city, county, precinct, neighborhood or other unit, would be needed in addition to, or be preferable to, the five-digit zip code.
In addition, to address concerns raised by commenters regarding access to birth date for research or other studies relating to young children or infants, the Department clarified that the Privacy Rule de-identification safe harbor allows disclosure of the age of an individual, including age expressed in months, days, or hours. Given that **the limited data s**et could include all ages, including age in months, days, or hours (if preferable), the Department requested comment on whether date of birth would be needed and, if so, whether the entire date would be needed, or just the month and year.
In addition, to further protect privacy, the Department proposed to condition the disclosure of the limited data set on covered entities obtaining from the recipients a data use or similar agreement, in which the recipient would agree to limit the use of the limited data set to the purposes specified in the Privacy Rule, to limit who can use or receive the data, and agree not to reidentify the data or contact the individuals.

17.4.3 Summary of the HIPAA Privacy Rule

(United States, Department of Health & Human Services, cf. (14))

The following identifiers of the individual or of relatives, employers, or household members of the individual must be removed to achieve the **"safe harbor" method of de-identification:**

(A) **Names**
(B) **All geographic subdivisions smaller than a State**,
including street address, city, county, precinct, zip code, and their equivalent geocodes, except for the initial three digits of a zip code if, according to the current publicly available data from the Bureau of Census
   (1) the geographic units formed by combining all zip codes with the same three initial digits contains more than 20,000 people; and
   (2) the initial three digits of a zip code for all such geographic units containing 20,000 or fewer people is changed to 000;

(C) **All elements of dates (except year)**
for dates directly related to the individual, including birth date, admission date, discharge date, date of death; and all ages over 89 and all elements of dates (including year) indicative of such age, except that such ages and elements may be aggregated into a single category of age 90 or older;
(D) **Telephone numbers;**
(E) **Fax numbers;**
(F) **Electronic mail addresses**:
(G) **Social security numbers;**
(H) **Medical record numbers;**
(I) **Health plan beneficiary numbers;**
(J) **Account numbers;**
(K) **Certificate/license numbers;**
(L) **Vehicle identifiers and serial numbers,**
including license plate numbers;
(M) **Device identifiers and serial numbers;**
(N) **Web Universal Resource Locators (URLs);**
(O) **Internet Protocol (IP) address numbers;**
(P) **Biometric identifiers,**
including finger and voice prints;
(Q) **Full face photographic images**
and any comparable images; and any other unique identifying number, characteristic, or code, except as permitted for re-identification purposes provided certain conditions are met In addition to the removal of the above-stated identifiers, the covered entity may not have actual knowledge that the remaining information could be used alone or in combination with any other information to identify an individual who is subject of the information. 45 C.F.R. § 164.514(b).

17.4.4 General Principles in the context health research

(involving personally identifiable data (cf. (42)))

The following principles are recommended for organizations that conduct, sponsor, or regulate health research involving personally identifiable data. They can be transposed into professional guidelines, standard operating principles, regulations, or laws. Criteria and procedures should be established that are specific to the context.

- *Overall in health research, cultivate an atmosphere of respect for the privacy of the people whose health experience is being studied.*
- *Collect or use personally identifiable data only if the research is worthwhile and identifiability is required for scientific reasons.*
- *Urge Institutional Review Boards and other ethics review bodies to become fully engaged with the privacy, confidentiality, and security aspects of subject protection, in secondary research on data as well as in direct experimentation.*
- *Respect such standard fair-use practices as announcing the existence of data collections, allowing data-subjects to review data about themselves, and the like. If for scientific reasons*

exceptions have to be made to normal practice, this should be discussed as part of the informed consent process before the study starts.
- *Attend sensitively to informing data subjects and gaining informed consent.*
- *Safeguard personal identifiers as close to the point of original data collection as possible.*
- *Enforce a policy of "No access to personally identifiable information" as the default – then base exceptional access on need-to-know.*
- *Generally limit the cordon-of-access to personally identifiable data. Allow access for formally justified research uses and to appropriate researchers. Maintain and monitor access "audit trails."*
- *Remove data-subjects' personal identifiability as thoroughly as is compatible with research needs. If key-coding, aggregating, or otherwise removing personally identifying information, do so with adequate rigor.*
- *Maintain proper physical safeguards and cybersecurity measures. Periodically challenge them, to test their adequacy.*
- *Develop policies on seeking or allowing secondary use of personally identifiable data, and on the associated conditions and safeguards.*
- *Before either (a) transferring data to other researchers or organizations, or (b) using data for new purposes, make conscientious decisions as to whether to proceed and what the privacy protections should be. Then if proceeding, implement appropriate protections.*
- *Sensitize, train, and certify all personnel who handle personally identifiable data or supervise those who do. Make data stewardship responsibilities clear. Promote internal and external accountability.*

18 Appendix 4: Informed Consent (IC)

18.1 The Nuremberg Code

DIRECTIVES FOR HUMAN EXPERIMENTATION
(Cf. http://www.nus.edu.sg/irb/Articles/Nuremberg.pdf)

The Nuremberg Military Tribunal's decision in the case of the United States vs. Karl Brandt et al. includes what is now called the Nuremberg Code, a ten point statement delimiting permissible medical experimentation on human subjects. According to this statement, humane experimentation is justified only if its results benefit society and it is carried out in accord with basic principles that "satisfy moral, ethical, and legal concepts." To some extent the Nuremberg Code has been superseded by the Declaration of Helsinki as a guide for human experimentation.

– "Permissible Medical Experiments." Trials of War Criminals before the Nuremberg Military Tribunals under Control Council Law No. 10. Nuremberg October 1946 – April 1949, Washington. U.S. Government Printing Office (n.d.), vol. 2., pp. 181-182.

1. The voluntary consent of the human subject is absolutely essential. This means that the person involved should have legal capacity to give consent; should be situated as to be able to exercise free power of choice, without the intervention of any element of force, fraud, deceit, duress, over-reaching, or other ulterior form of constraint or coercion, and should have sufficient knowledge and comprehension of the elements of the subject matter involved as to enable him to make an understanding and enlightened decision. This latter element requires that before the acceptance of an affirmative decision by the experimental subject there should be made known to him the nature, duration, and purpose of the experiment; the method and means by which it is to be conducted; all inconveniences and hazards reasonably to be expected; and the effects upon his health or person which may possibly come from his participation in the experiment.
   The duty and responsibility for ascertaining the quality of the consent rests upon each individual who initiates, directs or engages in the experiment. It is a personal duty and responsibility which may not be delegated to another with impunity.
2. The experiment should be such as to yield fruitful results for the good of society, unprocurable by other methods or means of study, and not random and unnecessary in nature.
3. The experiment should be so designed and based on the results of animal experimentation and a knowledge of the natural history of the disease or other problem under study that the anticipated results will justify the performance of the experiment.
4. The experiment should be so conducted as to avoid all unnecessary physical and mental suffering and injury.
5. No experiment should be conducted where there is an a priori reason to believe that death or disabling injury will occur; except, perhaps, in those experiments where the experimental physicians also serve as subjects.
6. The degree of risk to be taken should never exceed that determined by the humanitarian importance of the problem to be solved by the experiment.

7. Proper preparations should be made and adequate facilities provided to protect the experimental subject against even remote possibilities of injury disability or death.
8. The experiment should be conducted only by scientifically qualified persons. The highest degree of skill and care should be required through all stages of the experiment of those who conduct or engage in the experiment.
9. During the course of the experiment the human subject should be at liberty to bring the experiment to an end if he has reached the physical or mental state where continuation of the experiment seems to him to be impossible.
10. During the course of the experiment the scientist in charge must be prepared to terminate the experiment at any stage, if he has probable cause to believe, in the exercise of the good faith, superior skill and careful judgement required by him that a continuation of the experiment is likely to result in injury, disability, or death to the experimental subject.

18.2 EU Privacy Directive (October 24, 1995)

SECTION II – CRITERIA FOR MAKING DATA PROCESSING LEGITIMATE
Article 7

Member States shall provide that personal data may be processed only if:
(a) the data subject has unambiguously given his consent; or
(b) processing is necessary for the performance of a contract to which the data subject is party or in order to take steps at the request of the data subject prior to entering into a contract; or
(c) processing is necessary for compliance with a legal obligation to which the controller is subject; or
(d) processing is necessary in order to protect the vital interests of the data subject; or
(e) processing is necessary for the performance of a task carried out in the public interest or in the exercise of official authority vested in the controller or in a third party to whom the data are disclosed; or
(f) processing is necessary for the purposes of the legitimate interests pursued by the controller or by the third party or parties to whom the data are disclosed, except where such interests are overridden by the interests for fundamental rights and freedoms of the data subject which require protection under Article 1 (1).

SECTION III – SPECIAL CATEGORIES OF PROCESSING
Article 8

The processing of special categories of data
1. Member States shall prohibit the processing of personal data revealing racial or ethnic origin, political opinions, religious or philosophical beliefs, trade-union membership, and the processing of data concerning health or sex life.
2. Paragraph 1 shall not apply where:
    (a) the data subject has given his explicit consent to the processing of those data, except where the laws of the Member State provide that the prohibition referred to in paragraph 1 may not be lifted by the data subject's giving his consent; or
    (b) processing is necessary for the purposes of carrying out the obligations and specific rights of the controller in the field of employment law in so far as it is authorized by national law providing for adequate safeguards; or
    (c) processing is necessary to protect the vital interests of the data subject or of another person where the data subject is physically or legally incapable of giving his consent; or

(d) processing is carried out in the course of its legitimate activities with appropriate guarantees by a foundation, association or any other non-profit-seeking body with a political, philosophical, religious or trade-union aim and on condition that the processing relates solely to the members of the body or to persons who have regular contact with it in connection with its purposes and that the data are not disclosed to a third party without the consent of the data subjects; or

(e) the processing relates to data which are manifestly made public by the data subject or is necessary for the establishment, exercise or defence of legal claims.

3. Paragraph 1 shall not apply where processing of the data is required for the purposes of preventive medicine, medical diagnosis, the provision of care or treatment or the management of healthcare services, and where those data are processed by a health professsional subject under national law or rules established by national competent bodies to the obligation of professional secrecy or by another person also subject to an equivalent obligation of secrecy.

4. Subject to the provision of suitable safeguards, Member States may, for reasons of substantial public interest, lay down exemptions in addition to those laid down in paragraph 2 either by national law or by decision of the supervisory authority.

5. Processing of data relating to offences, criminal convictions or security measures may be carried out only under the control of official authority, or if suitable specific safeguards are provided under nationnal law, subject to derogations which may be granted by the Member State under national provisions providing suitable specific safeguards. However, a complete register of criminal convictions may be kept only under the control of official authority. Member States may provide that data relating to administrative sanctions or judgements in civil cases shall also be processed under the control of official authority.

6. Derogations from paragraph 1 provided for in paragraphs 4 and 5 shall be notified to the Commission.

7. Member States shall determine the condition under which a national identification number or any other identifier of general application may be processed.

18.3 COE – Rec No. R (97) 5, Explanatory Memorandum to Rec (97) 5

18.3.1 5. Information of the data subject

(COE – Recommendation No. R (97) 5, cf. (43) (44))

5.1. The data subject shall be informed of the following elements:
   a. the existence of a file containing his/her medical data and the type of data collected or to be collected;
   b. the purpose or purposes for which they are or will be processed;
   c. where applicable, the individuals or bodies from whom they are or will be collected;
   d. the persons or bodies to whom and the purposes for which they may be communicated;
   e. the possibility, if any, for the data subject to refuse his consent, to withdraw it and the consequences of such withdrawal;

f. the identity of the controller and of his/her representative, if any, as well as the conditions under which the rights of access and of rectification may be exercised.
5.2. The data subject should be informed at the latest at the moment of collection. However, when medical data are not collected from the data subject, the latter should be notified of the collection as soon as possible, as well as – in a suitable manner – of the information listed under Principle 5.1, unless this is clearly unreasonable or impracticable, or unless the data subject has already received the information.
5.3. Information for the data subject shall be appropriate and adapted to the circumstances. Information should preferably be given to each data subject individually.
5.4. Before a genetic analysis is carried out, the data subject should be informed about the objectives of the analysis and the possibility of unexpected findings.

Legally incapacitated persons
5.5. If the data subject is a legally incapacitated person, incapable of free decision and domestic law does not permit the data subject to act on his/her own behalf, the information shall be given to the person recognised as legally entitled to act in the interest of the data subject.
If a legally incapacitated person is capable of understanding, he/she should be informed before his/her data are collected or processed.

Some more explanations are given in Explanatory Memorandum to R (97) 5, (cf. (44))

114. The drafters of the recommendation underlined, however, that any relevant information, whether provided collectively or individually, is equally important, and should in all cases be appropriate.
115. The drafters of the recommendation also acknowledged that on some occasions the data subject may not have to be told some or all of the elements referred to in Principle 5.1, either because these elements are obvious to him/her from the context in which the medical data are collected, without the need for further explanation, or because he/she has already been properly informed of these elements on a previous occasion.
119. A genetic analysis may produce other results than the information sought; such unexpected findings, that is, findings which are not causally linked to the aim of the analysis, may cause harm to the data subject, or he/she might prefer not to know them. Moreover, the drafters of the recommendation felt that developments in genetic research are too recent and too significant to expect the uninitiated to be as familiar with the potential results as with those of a traditional medical examination. Principle 5.4 recommends therefore prior informing of the data subject on the objectives of the genetic analysis, and on the possibility of finding more. If necessary, this provision of information may be deferred.

18.3.2 6. Consent

(COE – Recommendation No. R (97) 5, cf. (43))

6.1. Where the data subject is required to give his/her consent, this consent should be free, express and informed.
6.2. The results of any genetic analysis should be formulated within the limits of the objectives of the medical consultation, diagnosis or treatment for which consent was obtained.

6.3. Where it is intended to process medical data relating to a legally incapacitated person who is incapable of free decision, and when domestic law does not permit the data subject to act on his/her own behalf, consent is required of the person recognised as legally entitled to act in the interest of the data subject or of an authority or any person or body provided for by law.
If, in accordance with Principle 5.5 above, a legally incapacitated person has been informed of the intention to collect or process his/her medical data, his/her wishes should be taken into account, unless domestic law provides otherwise.

Some more explanations are given in Explanatory Memorandum to R (97) 5, (cf. (44))

131. Consent is "informed" if the data subject is informed in particular of the purposes involved and the identity of the data controller. Consent is "free" if the data subject has the possibility to refuse his/her consent, to withdraw it or to modify the terms and conditions of consent.
136. Principle 6.2 provides that after genetic analysis the data subject should only be informed of the results in so far as these correspond to the objectives of the consultation, of the diagnosis, or of the treatment, unless the data subject himself/herself has asked for more information (see Principle 8.4 hereafter). In other words, the content of the consent is decisive for access to the results of the analysis (see paragraph 164 hereafter).

18.3.3 7. Communication

(COE – Recommendation No. R (97) 5, cf. (43))

7.1. Medical data shall not be communicated, unless on the conditions set out in this principle and in Principle 12.
7.2. In particular, unless other appropriate safeguards are provided by domestic law, medical data may only be communicated to a person who is subject to the rules of confidentiality incumbent upon a healthcare professional, or
to comparable rules of confidentiality, and who complies with the provisions of this recommendation

Some more explanations are given in Explanatory Memorandum to R (97) 5, (cf. (44))

143. It is obvious that medical data, one of the categories of sensitive data for which the convention requires special protection, should not be communicated outside the medical context in which they were collected, unless they are made anonymous (in which case the data no longer fall under the definition of personal data).

18.3.4 8. Rights of the data subject

(COE – Recommendation No. R (97) 5, cf. (43))

Rights of access and of rectification
8.1. Every person shall be enabled to have access to his/her medical data, either directly or through a healthcare professional or, if permitted by domestic law, a person appointed by him/her. The information must be accessible in understandable form.
8.2. Access to medical data may be refused, limited or delayed only if the law provides for this and if:
   a. this constitutes a necessary measure in a democratic society in the interests of protecting state security, public safety, or the suppression of criminal offences; or
   b. knowledge of the information is likely to cause serious harm to the data subject's health; or
   c. the information on the data subject also reveals information on third parties or if, with respect to genetic data, this information is likely to cause serious harm to consanguine or uterine kin or to a person who has a direct link with this genetic line; or
   d. the data are used for statistical or for scientific research purposes where there is clearly no risk of an infringement of the privacy of the data subject, notably the possibility of using the data collected in support of decisions or measures regarding any particular individual.
8.3. The data subject may ask for rectification of erroneous data concerning him/her and, in case of refusal, he/she shall be able to appeal.

Unexpected findings
8.4. The person subjected to genetic analysis should be informed of unexpected findings if the following conditions are met:
   a. domestic law does not prohibit the giving of such information;
   b. the person himself has asked for this information;
   c. the information is not likely to cause serious harm:
      i. to his/her health; or
      ii. to his/her consanguine or uterine kin, to a member of his/her social family, or to a person who has a direct link with his/her genetic line, unless domestic law provides other appropriate safeguards.
   Subject to sub-paragraph a, the person should also be informed if this information is of direct importance to him/her for treatment or prevention.

Some more explanations are given in Explanatory Memorandum to R (97) 5, (cf. (44))

153. One of the most important principles in the field of data protection, confirmed in Article 8 of the convention, is the right of every person to know the information about him/her stored by other persons. In the medical field there are three main obstacles to the application of this principle. Firstly, it may be extremely detrimental to the treatment of a patient if he/she is given the full facts about his/her case. Secondly, medical information as such may make little sense to the layman. And thirdly, medical data, and in particular genetic data, may concern also persons other than the data subject.

18.3 COE – Rec No. R (97) 5, Explanatory Memorandum to Rec (97) 5

Rights of access and rectification

154. Principle 8.1 summarises, in respect of medical data, the provisions under Article 8, paragraphs a and b, of the convention: as a general rule, every person shall be enabled to have access to information about himself/herself in a medical file and implicitly to know of its existence. Exceptions to this rule should be reduced to a minimum; as an example of such an exception, it might be detrimental for a patient to know that he/she is on record in a cancer register.

For this reason, Principle 8.1 leaves the option that the right of access be exercised indirectly (see the following paragraph); in that case, and unless this would be contrary to domestic law, the data subject should specify this and be enabled to designate for this purpose a person of his/her choice, who should be given full access.

Unexpected Findings

167. As indicated in paragraphs 119 and 160 above, unexpected results of a genetic analysis may cause harm to the data subject or other members of the genetic line which is of more importance than the data subject's right to know his/her own genetic data, for example, presence of unexpected family relations, or absence of presumed family relations. Such incidental data were not the purpose of the analysis; nobody asked for them. Moreover, Article 5 of the convention requires that data undergoing automatic processing shall be adequate, relevant and non-excessive. The best protection of such incidental data would be their immediate erasure.

168. Paragraph c of Principle 8.2 allows access to genetic data to be refused, limited or delayed, if it is provided for by law, if revealing these data is likely to cause serious harm to consanguine/uterine kin or to a person in the direct genetic line (see paragraph 160 above).

169. However, the drafters of the recommendation were aware that the convention also requires in Article 8 that the data subject shall be enabled to have access to his/her data. In the genetics sector, the right of access to probably complex data should be understood rather as a right to comprehensible information for the data subject. Moreover, it was noted that Principle 11 of Recommendation No. R (92) 3 on genetic testing and screening for healthcare purposes was worded as follows:

"In conformity with national legislation, unexpected findings may be communicated to the person tested only if they are of direct clinical importance to the person or the family. Communication of unexpected findings to family members of the person tested should only be authorised by national law if the person tested refuses expressly to release information even though the life of the family members is in danger."

18.3.5 12. Scientific Research

(COE – Recommendation No. R (97) 5, cf. (43))

12.1. Whenever possible, medical data used for scientific research purposes should be anonymous. Professional and scientific organisations as well as public authorities should promote the development of techniques and procedures securing anonymity.

12.2. However, if such anonymisation would make a scientific research project impossible, and the project is to be carried out for legitimate purposes, it could be carried out with personal data on condition that:

a. the data subject has given his/her informed consent for one or more research purposes; or
b. when the data subject is a legally incapacitated person incapable of free decision, and domestic law does not permit the data subject to act on his/her own behalf, his/her legal representative or an authority, or any person or body provided for by law, has given his/her consent in the framework of a research project related to the medical condition or illness of the data subject; or
c. disclosure of data for the purpose of a defined scientific research project concerning an important public interest has been authorised by the body or bodies designated by domestic law, but only if:
   i. the data subject has not expressly opposed disclosure; and
   ii. despite reasonable efforts, it would be impracticable to contact the data subject to seek his consent; and
   iii. the interests of the research project justify the authorisation; or
d. the scientific research is provided for by law and constitutes a necessary measure for public health reasons.

Some more explanations are given in Explanatory Memorandum to R (97) 5, (cf. (44))

Scientific research based on medical data
197. Although the recommendation does not refer to it explicitly, the requirement in Article 5 of the convention that personal data undergoing automatic processing should be adequate, relevant and not excessive applies equally to medical research: only the data necessary for the purposes of such research should be used.
198. The primary means of protecting medical data to be used for scientific research purposes, called for in Principle 12.1, is to make them anonymous. For this reason, researchers as well as public authorities concerned are urged to develop anonymisation techniques.
199. The second means of protection advocated by the recommendation involves arrangements for supervising planned research projects based on the quality requirements laid down in Article 5.b and 5.c of the convention (Principle 12.4; see paragraphs 211-212 hereafter).

18.4 Oviedo Convention

Convention for the Protection of Human Rights and Dignity of the Human Being with regard to the Application of Biology and Medicine: Convention on Human Rights and Biomedicine, European Treaty Series – No. 164, Oviedo, 4.IV.1997 (cf. (32))

Chapter II – Consent

Article 5 – General rule
An intervention in the health field may only be carried out after the person concerned has given free and informed consent to it.
This person shall beforehand be given appropriate information as to the purpose and nature of the intervention as well as on its consequences and risks. The person concerned may freely withdraw consent at any time.

Article 6 – Protection of persons not able to consent
1   Subject to Articles 17 and 20 below, an intervention may only be carried out on a person who does not have the capacity to consent, for his or her direct benefit.
2   Where, according to law, a minor does not have the capacity to consent to an intervention, the intervention may only be carried out with the authorisation of his or her representative or an authority or a person or body provided for by law.
    The opinion of the minor shall be taken into consideration as an increasingly determining factor in proportion to his or her age and degree of maturity.
3   Where, according to law, an adult does not have the capacity to consent to an intervention because of a mental disability, a disease or for similar reasons, the intervention may only be carried out with the authorisation of his or her representative or an authority or a person or body provided for by law.
    The individual concerned shall as far as possible take part in the authorisation procedure.
4   The representative, the authority, the person or the body mentioned in paragraphs 2 and 3 above shall be given, under the same conditions, the information referred to in Article 5.
5   The authorisation referred to in paragraphs 2 and 3 above may be withdrawn at any time in the best interests of the person concerned.

Article 7 – Protection of persons who have a mental disorder
Subject to protective conditions prescribed by law, including supervisory, control and appeal procedures, a person who has a mental disorder of a serious nature may be subjected, without his or her consent, to an intervention aimed at treating his or her mental disorder only where, without such treatment, serious harm is likely to result to his or her health.

18.5 UNESCO Universal Declaration on Bioethics and Human Rights

(UNESCO Universal Declaration on Bioethics and Human Rights of 2005, cf. (39))

Article 2 Aims
The aims of this Declaration are:
(a) to provide a universal framework of principles and procedures to guide States in the formulation of their legislation, policies or other instruments in the field of bioethics;
(b) to guide the actions of individuals, groups, communities, institutions and corporations, public and private;
(c) to promote respect for human dignity and protect human rights, by ensuring respect for the life of human beings, and fundamental freedoms, consistent with international human rights law;

Article 6 Consent
1. Any preventive, diagnostic and therapeutic medical intervention is only to be carried out with the prior, free and informed consent of the person concerned, based on adequate information. The consent should, where appropriate, be express and may be withdrawn by the person concerned at any time and for any reason without disadvantage or prejudice.
2. Scientific research should only be carried out with the prior, free, express and informed consent of the person concerned. The information should be adequate, provided in a comprehensible form and should include modalities for withdrawal of consent. Consent may

be withdrawn by the person concerned at any time and for any reason without any disadvantage or prejudice. Exceptions to this principle should be made only in accordance with ethical and legal standards adopted by States, consistent with the principles and provisions set out in this Declaration, in particular in Article 27, and international human rights law.
3. In appropriate cases of research carried out on a group of persons or a community, additional agreement of the legal representatives of the group or community concerned may be sought. In no case should a collective community agreement or the consent of a community leader or other authority substitute for an individual's informed consent.

Article 7 Persons without the capacity to consent
In accordance with domestic law, special protection is to be given to persons who do not have the capacity to consent:
(a) authorization for research and medical practice should be obtained in accordance with the best interest of the person concerned and in accordance with domestic law. However, the person concerned should be involved to the greatest extent possible in the decision-making process of consent, as well as that of withdrawing consent;
(b) research should only be carried out for his or her direct health benefit, subject to the authorization and the protective conditions prescribed by law, and if there is no research alternative of comparable effectiveness with research participants able to consent. Research which does not have potential direct health benefit should only be undertaken by way of exception, with the utmost restraint, exposing the person only to a minimal risk and minimal burden and if the research is expected to contribute to the health benefit of other persons in the same category, subject to the conditions prescribed by law and compatible with the protection of the individual's human rights. Refusal of such persons to take part in research should be respected.

Article 9 Privacy and confidentiality
The privacy of the persons concerned and the confidentiality of their personal information should be respected. To the greatest extent possible, such information should not be used or disclosed for purposes other than those for which it was collected or consented to, consistent with international law, in particular international human rights law.

18.6 Key Issues in Informed Consent for Pharmacogenomics Research

(Elements of informed consent for pharmacogenetic research; perspective of the pharmacogenetics working group, cf. (36))

The key issues of informed consent, as summarized by Julio Licinio and Ma-Li Wong, UCLA Laboratory for Pharmacogenomics, are given below.

(cf. Informed Consent in Pharmacogenomics, the Pharmacogenomics Journal (2002) 2, 343.)

- Early availability of the consent document permitting subjects to read it ahead of time, so that they can reflect and formulate questions prior to meeting for IC signature.
- Trained staff, fluent in the patients' language, who are available at the time of IC document signing and afterwards for answering questions.

18.6 Key Issues in Informed Consent for Pharmacogenomics Research

- *Description of sample collection.*
- *Is the same IC document used for the drug trial and for the pharmacogenomic study?*
- *Nature of association with drug trial: can one participate in the drug trial without donating DNA for the related pharmacogenomic study?*
- *Archiving DNA.*
- *Creation and immortalization of cell lines.*
- *Description of sample storage.*
- *Procedures for assurance of confidentiality.*
- *Description of the level of sample anonymity (samples can be identified, coded, double-coded/ de-identified, anonymized, or anonymous).*
- *Availability of procedures for withdrawing subjects' data and samples if they so desire at a later date and a clear description of the limitation to this approach, including timeline (e.g., once samples are anonymized it is no longer possible to retrieve them; once data are pooled, analyzed and presented or published it is no longer possible to retrieve them).*
- *Scientific use of the sample: can the sample be used only for the testing of a specific target/ hypothesis, or can it be used for any type of genetic or pharmacogenetic research?*
- *Ownership of the sample.*
- *Commercial uses of the sample (intellectual property).*
- *Distribution of genetic material to secondary users (even if the parties are not yet defined).*
- *Criteria for the distribution of genetic material to secondary users.*
- *Location of secondary users (national vs international).*
- *Type of primary or secondary users (academic, not-for-profit, for profit/-commercial).*
- *Compensation to subjects, if any.*
- *Personal vs society benefits.*
- *Options for contacting subjects in the future (possible only for non-anonymized/anonymous samples).*
- *Post-testing options for communication and sharing of genetic results with subjects.*
- *Sharing of unintended genetic results, particularly if directly relevant to medical care, with subjects, family members, or healthcare providers.*

18.7 International Declaration On Human Genetic Data

(for more details, cf. (4))

B. COLLECTION

Article 8: Consent
(a) Prior, free, informed and express consent, without inducement by financial or other personal gain, should be obtained for the collection of human genetic data, human proteomic data or biological samples, whether through invasive or non-invasive procedures, and for their subsequent processing, use and storage, whether carried out by public or private institutions. Limitations on this principle of consent should only be prescribed for compelling reasons by domestic law consistent with the international law of human rights.
(b) When, in accordance with domestic law, a person is incapable of giving informed consent, authorization should be obtained from the legal representative, in accordance with domestic law. The legal representative should have regard to the best interest of the person concerned.
(c) An adult not able to consent should as far as possible take part in the authorization procedure. The opinion of a minor should be taken into consideration as an increasingly determining factor in proportion to age and degree of maturity.
(d) In diagnosis and health care, genetic screening and testing of minors and adults not able to consent will normally only be ethically acceptable when it has important implications for the health of the person and has regard to his or her best interest.

Article 9: Withdrawal of consent
(a) When human genetic data, human proteomic data or biological samples are collected for medical and scientific research purposes, consent may be withdrawn by the person concerned unless such data are irretrievably unlinked to an identifiable person. In accordance with the provisions of Article 6(d), withdrawal of consent should entail neither a disadvantage nor a penalty for the person concerned.
(b) When a person withdraws consent, the person's genetic data, proteomic data and biological samples should no longer be used unless they are irretrievably unlinked to the person concerned.
(c) If not irretrievably unlinked, the data and biological samples should be dealt with in accordance with the wishes of the person. If the person's wishes cannot be determined or are not feasible or are unsafe, the data and biological samples should either be irretrievably unlinked or destroyed.

Article 10: The right to decide whether or not to be informed about research results
When human genetic data, human proteomic data or biological samples are collected for medical and scientific research purposes, the information provided at the time of consent should indicate that the person concerned has the right to decide whether or not to be informed of the results. This does not apply to research on data irretrievably unlinked to identifiable persons or to data that do not lead to individual findings concerning the persons who have participated in such a research. Where appropriate, the right not to be informed should be extended to identified relatives who may be affected by the results.

Article 11: Genetic counselling
It is ethically imperative that when genetic testing that may have significant implications for a person's health is being considered, genetic counselling should be made available in an appro-

priate manner. Genetic counselling should be non-directive, culturally adapted and consistent with the best interest of the person concerned.

Article 12: Collection of biological samples for forensic medicine or in civil, criminal and other legal proceedings
When human genetic data or human proteomic data are collected for the purposes of forensic medicine or in civil, criminal and other legal proceedings, including parentage testing, the collection of biological samples, in vivo or post-mortem, should be made only in accordance with domestic law consistent with the international law of human rights.

18.8 CIOMS – Ethical Guidelines for Biomedical Research

International Ethical Guidelines for Biomedical Research Involving Human Subjects, prepared by the Council for International Organizations of Medical Sciences (CIOMS) in collaboration with the World Health Organization (WHO), (cf. (37) and (38))

Guideline 5:
Obtaining informed consent: Essential information for prospective research subjects
Before requesting an individual's consent to participate in research, the investigator must provide the following information, in language or another form of communication that the individual can understand:
1. that the individual is invited to participate in research, the reasons for considering the individual suitable for the research, and that participation is voluntary;
2. that the individual is free to refuse to participate and will be free to withdraw from the research at any time without penalty or loss of benefits to which he or she would otherwise be entitled;
3. the purpose of the research, the procedures to be carried out by the investigator and the subject, and an explanation of how the research differs from routine medical care;
4. for controlled trials, an explanation of features of the research design (e.g.,randomization, double-blinding), and that the subject will not be told of the assigned treatment until the study has been completed and the blind has been broken;
5. the expected duration of the individual's participation (including number and duration of visits to the research centre and the total time involved) and the possibility of early termination of the trial or of the individual s participation in it;
6. whether money or other forms of material goods will be provided in return for the individual's participation and, if so, the kind and amount;
7. that, after the completion of the study, subjects will be informed of the findings of the research in general, and individual subjects will be informed of any finding that relates to their particular health status;
8. that subjects have the right of access to their data on demand, even if these data lack immediate clinical utility (unless the ethical review committee has approved temporary or permanent non-disclosure of data, in which case the subject should be informed of, and given, the reasons for such nondisclosure);
9. any foreseeable risks, pain or discomfort, or inconvenience to the individual (or others) associated with participation in the research, including risks to the health or well-being of a subject's spouse or partner;

10. the direct benefits, if any, expected to result to subjects from participating in the research
11. the expected benefits of the research to the community or to society at large, or contributions to scientific knowledge;
12. whether, when and how any products or interventions proven by the research to be safe and effective will be made available to subjects after they have completed their participation in the research, and whether they will be expected to pay for them;
13. any currently available alternative interventions or courses of treatment;
14. the provisions that will be made to ensure respect for the privacy of subjects and for the confidentiality of records in which subjects are identified;
15. the limits, legal or other, to the investigators' ability to safeguard confidentiality, and the possible consequences of breaches of confidentiality;
16. policy with regard to the use of results of genetic tests and familial genetic information, and the precautions in place to prevent disclosure of the results of a subject's genetic tests
17. to immediate family relatives or to others (e.g. insurance companies or employers) without the consent of the subject;
18. the sponsors of the research, the institutional affiliation of the investigators, and the nature and sources of funding for the research;
19. the possible research uses, direct or secondary, of the subject's medical records and of biological specimens taken in the course of clinical care (See also Guidelines 4 and 18 Commentaries);
20. whether it is planned that biological specimens collected in the research will be destroyed at its conclusion, and, if not, details about their storage (where, how, for how long, and final disposition) and possible future use, and that subjects have the right to decide about such future use, to refuse storage, and to have the material destroyed (See Guideline 4 Commentary);
21. whether commercial products may be developed from biological specimens, and whether the participant will receive monetary or other benefits from the development of such products;
22. whether the investigator is serving only as an investigator or as both investigator and the subject's physician;
23. the extent of the investigator's responsibility to provide medical services to the participant;
24. that treatment will be provided free of charge for specified types of research related injury or for complications associated with the research, the nature and duration of such care, the name of the organization or individual that will provide the treatment, and whether there is any uncertainty regarding funding of such treatment.
25. in what way, and by what organization, the subject or the subject's family or dependants will be compensated for disability or death resulting from such injury (or, when indicated, that there are no plans to provide such compensation);
26. whether or not, in the country in which the prospective subject is invited to participate in research, the right to compensation is legally guaranteed;
27. that an ethical review committee has approved or cleared the research protocol.

18.9 Human Genetic Examination Act (Genetic Diagnosis Act – GenDG)

Bundesrat Printed Matter 374/09 April 24, 2009 (cf. (40))

§ 8 **Consent**
(1) Any genetic examination or analysis may only be conducted, and any genetic sample may only be acquired for such a purpose, after the responsible medical person has received the express, written consent of the subject person, both in regard to the respective genetic examination and genetic sample. The consent stated in the foregoing sentence includes the decision in regard to the scope of the given genetic examination as well as regarding the decisions if, and if so to which extent, the examination results may be disclosed or, as the case may be, destroyed. A person or institution authorized according to § 7 (2) may only conduct any genetic analysis given proof of consent.
(2) The subject person may at any time with future effect revoke his or her permission vis-à-vis the responsible medical person either orally or in writing. Any oral revocation must be immediately documented. The responsible medical person must immediately transmit a copy of the proof of revocation of consent to the person or institution commissioned or authorized according to § 7 (2).

§ 9 **Duty to Inform**
(1) Before obtaining the subject person's consent the responsible medical person must first inform the subject person regarding the nature, meaning and scope or the genetic examination. The subject person must receive sufficient time for consideration before deciding to provide consent.
(2) In particular, the duty to inform includes
   1. clarification in regard to the purpose, type, scope and signifycance of the genetic examination including, without limitation, the achievable results given the proposed genetic study materials within the framework of the subject genetic examination; the foregoing also includes any genetic characteristics which are to be examined and which are significant in terms of avoiding, preventing or treating any illness or health condition,
   2. clarification of any health risks for the subject person in relation to gaining knowledge of the results of the subject genetic examination or gaining the genetic samples necessary thereto, including in the case of pregnant women clarification of any risks to the embryo or foetus related to conducting the genetic examination and gaining the necessary genetic samples,
   3. clarification as to the intended use of any genetic samples as well as the results of any genetic examinations or analyses,
   4. clarification of the right of any subject person to revoke his or her consent at any time,
   5. clarification in regard to the right of any subject person to not have to know results, including without limitation the right of the subject person to not have examination results, either partially or entirely, disclosed but to have them destroyed instead,
   6. in the case of a mass genetic screening, clarifying the subject person concerning the results of the evaluation of the examination undertaken by the Genetic Diagnostic Commission pursuant to § 16 (2).
(3) The responsible medical person must document the contents of each clarification before conducting the genetic examination.

§ 10 **Genetic Counselling**
(1) In the case of a diagnostic genetic examination, upon determination of the examination results, the responsible medical person shall offer the subject person counselling services performed by a medical doctor who fulfils the qualifications set forth in § 7(1) and § 7 (3). Should in the course of such examination a genetic characteristic of the subject person be determined with significance for an illness which according to the generally accepted status of science and technology is considered untreatable, then the foregoing sentence shall apply with the condition that the responsible medical person must offer counselling.
(2) In the case of a predictive genetic examination, counselling shall be offered to the subject person by a medical doctor who fulfils the qualifications set forth in § 7(1) and § 7 (3) to the extent that, on a case-by-case basis, the subject person has not after receiving written information detailing the contents of the genetic counselling waived such genetic counselling in writing. After counselling up until the examination, the affected person must receive appropriate time for consideration.
(3) Genetic counselling shall take place in a manner that is generally comprehendible and non-directive. In particular, it shall include a thorough explanation of possible medical, psychological and social issues which might arise in relation to conducting or, as the case may be, not conducting the subject genetic examination and as regards any given or potential examination results, alongside the possibilities of supporting the subject person in the context of any physical or psychological difficulties which have or may occur as a result of such genetic examination or its results. Given the consent of the subject person, an additional expert professional may be consulted. If it can be assumed that genetic relatives of the subject person are also carriers of the subject genetic characteristics with significance for an avoidable or treatable illness or health condition, genetic counselling shall include the recommendation that such relatives also undergo genetic counselling. Should the genetic examination be conducted on an embryo or foetus, the fourth sentence above applies accordingly.
(4) The responsible medical person who offered or conducted the genetic counselling must document its contents.

§ 11 **Reporting the Results of Genetic Examinations and Analyses**
(1) Subject to the conditions of Subparagraph (2) and Subparagraph (3), the result of any genetic examination may only be disclosed to the subject person and in each instance may only be disclosed by the responsible medical doctor or by the medical doctor who conducted the subject genetic counselling.
(2) Any person or institution authorized according to § 7 (2) to conduct genetic analyses may only disclose the results of such analyses to the medical person who commissioned the analyses.
(3) The responsible medical person may only disclose the results of any genetic examination or analysis with the express, written consent of the subject person.
(4) The results of any genetic analysis may not be disclosed to the extent the subject person has decided that the results of the given genetic examination shall be destroyed or where such person has revoked consent according to § 8 (2).

§ 12 **Retention and Destruction of Results of Genetic examinations and Analyses**
(1) The responsible medical person must retain the results of any genetic examinations and analyses of the subject person for a period of ten years. The responsible medical person must immediately destroy the genetic examinations and analyses contained in the examination records of the subject person
   1. if the retention period which is set forth in the first sentence has expired,

2. to the extent that the subject person has decided according to § 8 (1), first sentence, that the results of the given genetic examinations and analyses must be destroyed. To the extent that there is reason to believe that such destruction would infringe against the subject person's protected interests, or in cases where the subject person has requested in writing that the subject items be retained for a longer period of time, then instead of destroying the items pursuant to second sentence, Nr. 1, the responsible medical person must seal the results and must inform the person or institution authorized according to § 7 (2) thereof immediately.

(2) Subparagraph (1) applies accordingly to the retention, destruction or sealing of the results of genetic examinations conducted by persons or institutions authorized according to § 7 (2).

§ 13 Usage and Destruction of Genetic Samples

(1) Genetic samples may only be used for the purposes for which they were gained. As soon as any genetic sample is no longer required for such purposes, or the subject person has revoked consent according to § 8 (2), the responsible medical person or, as the case may be, the person or institution authorized according to § 7 (2) must immediately destroy the subject genetic sample.

(2) Genetic samples may only be used for other purposes that depart from

(1) to the extent that such use is permitted by other legal regulations or in cases where the person from whom the respective genetic sample stems has, after being fully informed in regard to the intended other purposes, provided express, written consent thereto.

(3) Anyone making use of a genetic sample must take all necessary technical and organizational measures to prevent any prohibited use of such sample.

§ 14 Genetic Examinations Involving Persons Lacking the Full Capacity to Consent

(1) In the case of any person who does not possess the capacity to recognize the nature, meaning or scope of a genetic examination, and is therefore unable to adjust his or her will accordingly, genetic examinations for medical purposes as well as gaining any genetic samples necessary therefore may only be conducted if

1. according to the generally accepted status of science and technology, doing so is necessary to avoid, prevent or treat a genetically-caused illness or health condition of the subject person, or if treatment with medication, which can affect genetic characteristics.
2. before proceeding the examination was explained

etc.

19 Appendix 5: Security

19.1 EU Privacy Directive (October 24, 1995)

Article 17: Security of Processing
1. Member States shall provide that the controller must implement appropriate technical and organizational measures to protect personal data against accidental or unlawful destruction or accidental loss, alteration, unauthorized disclosure or access, in particular where the processing involves the transmission of data over a network, and against all other unlawful forms of processing.
Having regard to the state of the art and the cost of their implementation, such measures shall ensure a level of security appropriate to the risks represented by the processing and the nature of the data to be protected.
2. The Member States shall provide that the controller must, where processing is carried out on his behalf, choose a processor providing sufficient guarantees in respect of the technical security measures and organizational measures governing the processing to be carried out, and must ensure compliance with those measures.
3. The carrying out of processing by way of a processor must be governed by a contract or legal act binding the processor to the controller and stipulating in particular that
the processor shall act only on instructions from the controller,
the obligations set out in paragraph 1, as defined by the law of the
Member State in which the processor is established, shall also be incumbent on the processor.
4. For the purposes of keeping proof, the parts of the contract or the legal act relating to data protection and the requirements relating to the measures referred to in paragraph 1 shall be in writing or in another equivalent form.

19.2 Federal Data Protection Act (Germany)

(Annex to the first sentence of Section 9, 1 January 2003)

Where personal data are processed or used automatically, the internal organization of authorities or enterprises is to be arranged in such a way that it meets the specific requirements of data protection. In particular, measures suited to the type of personal data or data categories to be protected shall be taken,

1. to prevent unauthorised persons from gaining access to data processing systems with which personal data are processed or used (access control),
2. to prevent data processing systems from being used without authorisation (access control),
3. to ensure that persons entitled to use a data processing system have access only to the data to which they have a right of access, and that personal data cannot be read, copied, modified or removed without authorisation in the course of processing or use and after storage (access control),
4. to ensure that personal data cannot be read, copied, modified or removed without authorisation during electronic transmission or transport, and that it is possible to check and

establish to which bodies the transfer of personal data by means of data transmission facilities is envisaged (transmission control),
5. to ensure that it is possible to check and establish whether and by whom personal data have been input into data processing systems, modified or removed (input control),
6. to ensure that, in the case of commissioned processing of personal data, the data are processed strictly in accordance with the instructions of the principal (job control),
7. to ensure that personal data are protected from accidental destruction or loss (availability control),
8. to ensure that data collected for different purposes can be processed separately.

19.3 Council of Europe Recommendation No. R (97) 5

3. Respect for privacy
3.1. The respect of rights and fundamental freedoms, and in particular of the right to privacy, shall be guaranteed during the collection and processing of medical data.
3.2. Medical data may only be collected and processed if in accordance with appropriate safeguards which must be provided by domestic law.

4. Collection and processing of medical data
4.1. Medical data shall be collected and processed fairly and lawfully and only for specified purposes.

9. Security
9.1. Appropriate **technical** and **organisational measures** shall be taken **to protect personal data** – processed in accordance with this recommendation – against accidental or illegal destruction, accidental loss, as well as against unauthorised access, alteration, communication or any other form of processing.
Such measures shall ensure an appropriate level of security taking account, on the one hand, of the technical state of the art and, on the other hand, of the sensitive nature of medical data and the evaluation of potential risks.
These measures shall be reviewed periodically.
9.2. In order to ensure in particular the confidentiality, integrity and accuracy of processed data, as well as the protection of patients, appropriate measures should be taken:
   a. to prevent any unauthorised person from having access to installations used for processing personal data (control of the entrance to installations);
   b. to prevent data media from being read, copied, altered or removed by unauthorised persons (control of data media);
   c. to prevent the unauthorised entry of data into the information system, and any unauthorised consultation, modification or deletion of processed personal data (memory control);
   d. to prevent automated data processing systems from being used by unauthorised persons by means of data transmission equipment (control of utilisation);
   e. with a view to, on the one hand, selective access to data and, on the other hand, the security of the medical data, to ensure that the processing as a general rule is so designed as to enable the separation of:
      – identifiers and data relating to the identity of persons;
      – administrative data;

- medical data;
- social data;
- genetic data (access control);

    f. to guarantee the possibility of checking and ascertaining to which persons or bodies personal data can be communicated by data transmission equipment (control of communication);

    g. to guarantee that it is possible to check and establish a posteriori who has had access to the system and what personal data have been introduced into the information system, when and by whom (control of data introduction);

    h. to prevent the unauthorised reading, copying, alteration or deletion of personal data during the communication of personal data and the transport of data media (control of transport);

    i. to safeguard data by making security copies (availability control).

9.3. Controllers of medical files should, in accordance with domestic law, draw up appropriate internal regulations which respect the related principles in this recommendation.

9.4. Where necessary, controllers of files processing medical data should appoint an independent person responsible for security of information systems and data protection and competent for giving advice on these issues.

19.4 US – Privacy Act of 1974 (Comments from William W. Lowrance, cf. (42))

Covers personally identifiable data held by the Federal government. The Privacy Act has been widely noted to have serious weaknesses, among them that:
- *It does not cover data held outside the Federal government.*
- *It covers only data about U.S. citizens and aliens permanently residing in the U.S., not data about citizens of other countries.*
- *Its "routine use" provision is lax.*
- *Few legal avenues are provided for citizens to seek injunctive or other relief if they believe their rights are being violated.*
- *Its protections do not continue after the death of the data subject.*

Basic security measures
Security has many dimensions. The challenge is to keep data sequestered and protect its integrity, but at the same time to keep it accessible for authorized users who have legitimate need to use it. In its provocative recent report on these issues, For the Record: Protecting Electronic Health Information, a committee of the National Research Council recommended immediate implementation of these technical practices and procedures:
- *Individual authentication of users.*
- *Access controls based on legitimate need-to-know.*
- *Audit trails (maintaining access logs).*
- *Physical security and disaster recovery (limiting physical access, carefully storing backup data).*
- *Protection of remote access points (controlling external access).*
- *Protection of external electronic communications (not sending personally identifiable data over public networks).*
- *Software discipline (virus-checking, controlling software installation).*

System assessment (testing security on an ongoing basis).

The committee also recommended adoption of these **organizational practices***:*
- *Security and confidentiality policies.*
- *Security and confidentiality committees.*
- *Information security officers.*
- *Education and training programs.*
- *Sanctions.*
- *Improved authorization forms.*

19.5 Safe Harbor Privacy Principles (2000)

Like many countries, the US have recently undertaken initiatives aimed at harmonizing national privacy standards with the provisions of the EU Privacy Directive. As noted in Section 10.3, above, Article 25 of the Directive generally prohibits the transfer of personal data from EU member nations to those lacking an "adequate level of protection." In the absence of a uniform or central data protection statute in the US, the US Department of Commerce has sought to institute standards that would enable US companies to be included in the transfer of personal information from Europe. Following some two years of de-liberations, negotiation and revision after an initial US proposal of 1999, the US and EU approved the final US Safe Harbor Privacy Framework89 in July 2000. The Framework consists of a number of documents from the US and the EU. The key documents include the US Department of Commerce's Safe Harbor Privacy Principles and the Frequently Asked Questions (FAQs).

19.6 UN – ICCPR International Covenant on Civil and Political Rights

The respect of privacy as a fundamental principle of international law was formally integrated into the broader international community in 1966, when the UN General Assembly adopted and opened for signature the **International Covenant on Civil and Political Rights (ICCPR)**.

Article 17
1. No one shall be subjected to arbitrary or unlawful interference with his privacy, family, or correspondence, nor to unlawful attacks on his honour and reputation.
2. Everyone has the right to the protection of the law against such interference or attacks.

20 Abbreviations

Anonymization

aCDB	anonymized Clinical Data Base
AGN	Aliquot Group Number
bSID	barcoded Sample Identifier
c	column of a rack
CDI	Clinical Data Identifier
CRF	Case Report Form
eCRF	electronic Case Report Form
CROSID	CRO Sample IDentifier
CTP	Clinical Trial Protocol
DPDB	Data Protection Data Base
GDI	Genetic Data Identifier
GRB	Genetic Review Board
	Company/Institution internal counterpart to Ethical Committee in the context of requests for common evaluations of anonymized clinical and related genetic data.
KPDB	Key Protection Data Base
nCDI	new Clinical Data Identifier
nGDI	new Genetic Data Identifier
nRackID	new Rack IDentifier
r	row of a rack
rCDI	request Clinical Data Identifier
rGDI	request Genetic Data Identifier
RackID	Rack IDentifier
RID	Random IDentifier
RPATID	Random PATient IDentifier
SDV	Source Data Verification
SEA	Secure Evaluation Area
SGN	Sample Group Number
SML	Sample Management/Lims
TCM	Trial Clinical Monitor

General

BCR	Binding Corporate Rules
BDSG	Bundes DatenSchutz Gesetz
	Federal data protection act of Germany
CFR	Code of Federal Regulations
CIOMS	Council for International Organizations of Medical Sciences
COE	Council Of Europe
DHHS	U.S. Department of Health and Human Services
DPA	Data Protection Authority
DPO	Data Protection Officer

EC	**E**thical **C**ommittee
ECHR	**E**uropean **C**onvention on **H**uman **R**ights and Fundamental Freedoms
EDPS	**E**uropean **D**ata **P**rotection **S**upervisor
EEA	**E**uropean **E**conomic **A**rea
EFTA	**E**uropean **F**ree **T**rade **A**ssociation
EHR	**E**lectronic **H**ealth **R**ecord
EMA	**E**uropean **M**edicines **A**gency
ETS	**E**uropean **T**reaty **S**eries
EU	**E**uropean **U**nion
EU Commission	**EU**ropean **Commission** makes proposals for the European Union legislation to the European Parliament and the Council of the European Union. In addition, it monitors the implementation of the legislation after adoption by the EU Council of Ministers.
FDA	**F**ood and **D**rug **A**dministration
FP7	**FP7** is the short name for the Seventh Framework Programme for Research and Technological Development. This is the EU's main instrument for funding research in Europe and it will run from 2007-2013. FP7 is also designed to respond to Europe's employment needs, competitiveness and quality of life.
GCP	**G**ood **C**linical **P**ractice
GINA	The U.S. **G**enetic **I**nformation **N**ondiscrimination **A**ct
HIPAA	**H**ealth **I**nsurance **P**ortability and **A**ccountability **A**ct
HIPAA Privacy Rule	Standards for Privacy of Individually Identifiable Health Information
IC	**I**nformed **C**onsent
ICCPR	**I**nternational **C**ovenant on **C**ivil and **P**olitical **R**ights
IQ	**I**nstallation **Q**ualification
IRB	**I**nstitutional **R**eview **B**oard
OECD	**O**rganisation for **E**conomic **C**o-operation and **D**evelopment
OHRP	U.S. **O**ffice of **H**uman **R**esearch **P**rotections
OQ	**O**perational **Q**ualification
PHS	U.S. **P**ublic **H**ealth **S**ervice
PQ	**P**erformance **Q**ualification
SCC	**S**tandard **C**ontractual **C**lauses
SDLC	**S**ystem **D**evelopment **L**ife **C**ycle
TFEU	**T**reaty on the **F**unctioning of the **E**uropean **U**nion
UNESCO	**U**nited **N**ations **E**ducational, **S**cientific and **C**ultural **O**rganization
WHO	**W**orld **H**ealth **O**rganization
WMA	**W**orld **M**edical **A**ssociation

21 References

1. EMEA, *ICH Topic E 6 (R1), Guideline for Good Clinical Practice*, 2002, July.
2. Deutscher Ethikrat, *Human biobanks for research*, 2010.
3. Deutscher Ethikrat, *Predictive health information in preemployment medical examinations*, 2005, Aug 16.
4. UNESCO, *International Declaration on Human Genetic*, 2003, Oct 16.
5. The Pharmacogenetics Working Group, *Terminology for sample collection in clinical genetic Studies, The Pharmacogenomics Journal (2001) 1, 101–103*, 2001.
6. EMEA, *Position Paper on Terminology in Pharmacogenetics*, 2002, Nov 21.
7. EMEA, *Understanding the Terminology used in Pharmacogenetics*, 2004, Jul 29.
8. B.M. Knoppers, M. Saginur, *The Babel of Genetic Data Terminology, Nature Biotechnology, Vol. 23 No. 8*, 2005, Aug.
9. B.M. Knoppers, *Population Biobanks Lexicon, Public Population Project in Genomics (P3G) & Promoting Harmonization of Epidemiological Biobanks in Europe (PHOEBE)*, 2007, Jul.
10. Instituto de Salud Carlos III, Madrid, *Outstanding legal and ethical issues on biobanks, an overview on the regulations of member states of the EuroBioBank project*, 2005.
11. Bernice S. Elger & Arthur L.Caplan, *Consent and anonymization in research involving biobanks, EMBO (European Molecular Biology Organization) reports Vol. 7, No. 7*, 2006.
12. DHHS (U.S. Department of Health and Human Services), *45 CFR Parts 160 and 164, Standards for Privacy of Individually Identifiable Health Information; Final Rule*, 2000, Dec 28.
13. OCR (U.S. Office for Civil Rights), *Summary of the HIPAA Privacy Rule*, 2003, May.
14. *Health Insurance Portability and Accountability Act of 1996, 104th Congress, Public Law 104–191*, 1996.
15. COE (Council Of Europe, Committee Of Ministers), *Recommendation No. R (92) 3 on Genetic Testing and Screening for Health Care Purposes*, 1992, Feb 10.
16. *Federal Data Protection Act (BDSG) (English and German version)*, 2006, Nov 15.
17. *Federal Data Protection Act (BDSG) in the version promulgated on 14 January 2003 (Federal Law Gazette I, p. 66), last amended by Article 1 of the Act of 14 August 2009 (Federal Law Gazette, 2009, Sep 1)*.
18. European Parliament and Council, *Directive 2001/20/EC on the approximation of the laws, regulations and administrative provisions of the Member States relating to the implementation of good clinical practice in the conduct of clinical trials on medicinal products for human use*, 2001, Apr 4.
19. Foundation for EU Democracy, *Consolidated Reader-Friendly Edition of the Treaty on European Union (TEU) and the Treaty on the Functioning of the European Union (TFEU) as amended by the Treaty of Lisbon (2007)*, 2008.
20. Christine Fretten, Vaughne Miller, *The European Union: a guide to terminology, procedures and sources, Standard Note: SN/IA/3689, House of Commons*, 2005, Jul 21.
21. COE (Council Of Europe), *Convention for the Protection of Human Rights and Fundamental Freedoms*, 1950, Nov 4.
22. *Charter of Fundamental Rights of the European Union, Official Journal of the European Communities*, 2000, Dec 18.
23. European Parliament and Council, *Directive 95/46/EC on the protection of individuals with regard to the processing of personal data and on the free movement of such data*, 1995, Oct 24. (remark: this directive is also referred to as EU Privacy Directive)
24. European Parliament and Council, *Directive 2002/58/EC concerning the processing of personal data and the protection of privacy in the electronic communications sector (Directive on privacy and electronic communications)*, 2002, Jul 12.

25. DHHS (U.S. Department of Health and Human Services), *45 CFR 46, Protection of Human Subjects (Common Rule)*, Federal Register, pp. 28003-28032, 1991, Jun 18.
26. GPO (U.S. Government Printing Office), *Genetic Information Nondiscrimination Act of 2008, an Act to prohibit discrimination on the basis of genetic information with respect to health insurance and employment*, Public Law 110–233, 2008, May 21.
27. DHHS (U.S. Department of Health and Human Services), *Guidance on the Genetic Information Nondiscrimination Act: Implications for Investigators and Institutional Review Boards*, Office for Human Research Protections (OHRP), 2009, Mar 24.
28. DHHS (U.S. Department of Health and Human Services), *"GINA" – The Genetic Information Nondiscrimination Act of 2008, Information for Researchers and Health Care Professionals*, 2009, Apr 6.
29. George J. Annas, Patricia (Winnie) Roche, Robert C. Green, *GINA, GENISM, and Civil Rights*, Bioethics, pp. ii-iv, 2008, Jul.
30. Kathy L. Hudson, Ph.D., M.K. Holohan, J.D., and Francis S. Collins, M.D., Ph.D., *Keeping Pace with the Times – The Genetic Information Nondiscrimination Act of 2008*, n engl j med, Vol. 358, 2008, Jun 19.
31. WMA (World Medical Association), *World Medical Association Declaration of Helsinki, Ethical Principles for Medical Research Involving Human Subjects*, 2008, Oct.
32. COE (Council Of Europe), *Convention for the Protection of Human Rights and Dignity of the Human Being with regard to the Application of Biology and Medicine: Convention on Human Rights and Biomedicine*, ETS No. 164, 1997, Apr 4.
33. DHHS (U.S. Department of Health and Human Services), *Code of Federal Regulations Title 45 Public Welfare, Part 46 Protection of Human Subjects (45 CFR 46)*, 2009, Jan 15.
34. DHHS (U.S. Department of Health and Human Services), *21 CFR Part 50 – Protection of Human Subjects*, 2002, Mar 15.
35. 62. Konferenz der Datenschutzbeauftragten des Bundes und der Länder, *Entschließung: Gesetzliche Regelung von genetischen Untersuchungen*, Münster/Westf., 2001, Oct 24-28.
36. DC Anderson et al on behalf of the Pharmacogenetics Working Group, *Elements of informed consent for pharmacogenetic research; perspective of the pharmacogenetics working group*, The Pharmacogenomics Journal, (2002) 2, pp. 284–292.
37. CIOMS (Council for International Organizations of Medical Sciences), WHO (World Health Organization), *International Ethical Guidelines for Biomedical Research Involving Human Subjects*, 2002.
38. CIOMS (Council for International Organizations of Medical Sciences), WHO (World Health Organization), *International Ethical Guidelines for Biomedical Research Involving Human Subjects*, Annex 2, 2005, Aug 9.
39. UNESCO (United Nations Educational, Scientific and Cultural Organization), *Universal Declaration on Bioethics and Human Rights*, 2005, Oct 19.
40. Bundesrat, *Enactment of the German Federal Parliament (Bundestag) Human Genetic Examination Act (Genetic Diagnosis Act – GenDG), during its 218th session on April 24, 2009*, 2009, Apr 24.
41. Spain, *Protection of Personal Data*, Organic Law 15, 1999, Dec 13.
42. William W. Lowrance, *Privacy and Health Research, A Report to the U.S. Secretary of Health and Human Services*, 1997, May.
43. COE (Council Of Europe, Committee Of Ministers), *Recommendation No. R (97) 5 on the Protection of Medical Data*, 1997, Feb 13.
44. COE (Council Of Europe, Committee Of Ministers), Explanatory Memorandum, R*ecommendation No. R (97) 5 on the Protection of Medical Data*, 1997, Feb 13.

45. European Parliament and Council, *Directive 97/66/EC concerning the processing of personal data and the protection of privacy in the telecommunications sector*, 1997, Dec 15.
46. Julio Licinio, Ma-Li Wong, *Informed Consent in Pharmacogenomics*, The Pharmacogenomics Journal, (2002) 2, 343.
47. COE (Council Of Europe), *Convention for the Protection of Individuals with Regard to Automatic Processing of Personal Data*, ETS No. 108, 1981, Jan 28.
48. European Parliament and the Council, *Regulation (EC) No 45/2001 on the protection of individuals with regard to the processing of personal data by the Community institutions and bodies and on the free movement of such data (2000, Dec 18)*, Official Journal of the European Communities, 2001, Jan 12.
49. Committee of Ministers (EU), *Recommendation No. R (81) 1, Regulations for automated medical data banks (including the Explanatory Memorandum)*, 1981, Jan 23.
50. Committee of Ministers (EU), *Recommendation No. R (83) 10, on the protection of personal data used for scientific research and statistics*, 1983, Sep 23.
51. Committee of Ministers (EU), *Explanatory Memorandum, Recommendation No. R (83) 10 on the protection of personal data used for scientific research and statistics*, 1983, Sep 23.
52. Committee of Ministers (EU), *Recommendation No. R (85) 20 on the protection of personal data used for the purposes of direct marketing*, 1985, Oct 25.
53. Committee of Ministers (EU), *Explanatory Memorandum, Recommendation No. R (85) 20 on the protection of personal data used for the purposes of direct marketing*, 1985, Oct 25.
54. Committee of Ministers (EU), *Recommendation No. R (86) 1 on the protection of personal data for social security purposes*, 1986, Jan 23.
55. Committee of Ministers (EU), *Explanatory Memorandum, Recommendation No. R (86) 1 on the protection of personal data for social security purposes*, 1986, Jan 23.
56. Committee of Ministers (EU), *Recommendation No. R (87) 15 regulating the use of personal data in the police sector*, 1987, Sep 17.
57. Project Group on Data Protection (CJ-PD), *First Evaluation of the Relevance of Recommendation No. R (87) 15 regulating the Use of Personal Data in the Police Sector*, 1994, Dec.
58. Project Group on Data Protection (CJ-PD), *Second Evaluation of the Relevance of Recommendation No. R (87) 15 regulating the Use of Personal Data in the Police Sector*, 1998, Dec.
59. Project Group on Data Protection (CJ-PD), *Report on the Third Evaluation of the Relevance of Recommendation No. R (87) 15 regulating the Use of Personal Data in the Police Sector*, 2002.
60. COE (Council Of Europe, Committee Of Ministers), *Recommendation No. R (89) 2 on the protection of personal data used for employment purposes*, 1989, Jan 18.
61. COE (Council Of Europe, Committee Of Ministers), *Explanatory Memorandum, Recommendation No. R (89) 2 concerning the protection of personal data used for employment purposes*, 1989, Jan 18.
62. COE (Council Of Europe, Committee Of Ministers), *Recommendation No. R (90) 19 on the protection of personal data used for payment and other related operations*, 1990, Sep 13.
63. COE (Council Of Europe, Committee Of Ministers), *Explanatory Memorandum, Recommendation No. R (90) 19 concerning the protection of personal data used for payment and other related operations*, 1990, Sep 13.
64. COE (Council Of Europe, Committee Of Ministers), *Recommendation No. R (91) 10 on the communication to third parties of personal data held by public bodies*, 1991, Sep 9.
65. COE (Council Of Europe, Committee Of Ministers), *Explanatory Memorandum, Recommendation No. R (91) 10 on the communication to third parties of personal data held by public bodies*, 1991, Sep 9.

66. COE (Council Of Europe, Committee Of Ministers), *Recommendation No. R (92) 1 on the use of analysis of Deoxyribonucleic Acid (DNA) within the framework of the criminal justice system*, 1992, Feb 10.
67. COE (Council Of Europe, Committee Of Ministers), *Recommendation No. R (95) 4 on the protection of personal data in the area of telecommunication services, with particular reference to telephone services*, 1995, Feb 7.
68. COE (Council Of Europe, Committee Of Ministers), *Explanatory Memorandum, Recommendation No. R (95) 4 on the protection of personal data in the area of telecommunication services, with particular reference to telephone services*, 1995, Feb 7.
69. COE (Council Of Europe, Committee Of Ministers), *Recommendation No. R (97) 18 concerning the protection of personal data collected and processed for statistical purposes*, 1997, Sep 30.
70. COE (Council Of Europe, Committee Of Ministers), *Explanatory Memorandum, Recommendation No. R (97) 18 concerning the protection of personal data collected and processed for statistical purposes*, 1997, Sep 30.
71. COE (Council Of Europe, Committee Of Ministers), *Recommendation No. R (99) 5 for the protection of privacy on the Internet*, 1999, Feb 23.
72. COE (Council Of Europe, Committee Of Ministers), *Recommendation Rec (2002) 9 on the protection of personal data collected and processed for insurance purposes*, 2002, Sep 18.
73. COE (Council Of Europe, Committee Of Ministers), *Explanatory Memorandum, Recommendation No. R (2002) 9 on the protection of personal data collected and processed for insurance purposes*, 2002, Sep 18.
74. COE (Council Of Europe, Committee Of Ministers), *Recommendation Rec (2006) 4, on research on biological Materials of Human Origin*, 2006, Mar 15.
75. Article 29 Data Protection Working Party, *WP4, Working Party on the Protection of Individuals With Regard to the Processing of Personal Data. First Orientations on Transfers of Personal Data to Third Countries – Possible Ways Forward in Assessing Adequacy*, 1997, Jun 26.
76. Article 29 Data Protection Working Party, *WP80, Working document on biometrics*, 2003, Aug 1.
77. Article 29 Data Protection Working Party, *WP91, Working Document on Genetic Data*, 2004, Mar 17.
78. Article 29 Data Protection Working Party, *WP114, Working document on a common interpretation of Article 26(1) of Directive 95/46/EC of 24 October 1995*, 2005, Nov 25.
79. Article 29 Data Protection Working Party, *WP131, Working Document on the processing of personal data relating to health in electronic health records (EHR)*, 2007, Feb 15.
80. Article 29 Data Protection Working Party, *WP136, Opinion 4/2007 on the concept of personal data*, 2007, Jun 20.
81. Article 29 Data Protection Working Party, *WP159, Opinion 1/2009 on the proposals amending Directive 2002/58/EC on privacy and electronic communications (e-Privacy Directive)*, 2009, Feb 10.
82. European Parliament and Council, *Directive 2006/24/EC on the retention of data generated or processed in connection with the provision of publicly available electronic communications services or of public communications networks and amending Directive 2002/58/EC*, 2006, Mar 15.
83. European Parliament and Council, *Directive 2001/83/EC on the Community code relating to medicinal products for human use*, 2001, Nov 6.
84. European Parliament and Council, *Directive 2002/98/EC setting standards of quality and safety for the collection, testing, processing, storage and distribution of human blood and blood components and amending Directive 2001/83/EC*, 2003, Jan 27.
85. Commission of the European Communities, *Commission Directive 2004/33/EC implementing Directive 2002/98/EC of the European Parliament and of the Council as regards certain*

technical requirements for blood and blood components (Text with EEA relevance), 2004, Mar 22.
86. European Parliament and Council, *Directive 2004/23/EC on setting standards of quality and safety for the donation, procurement, testing, processing, preservation, storage and distribution of human tissues and cells*, 2004, Mar 31.
87. Commission of the European Communities, *Commission Directive 2006/17/EC implementing Directive 2004/23/EC of the European Parliament and of the Council as regards certain technical requirements for the donation, procurement and testing of human tissues and cells (Text with EEA relevance)*, 2006, Feb 8.
88. Commission of the European Communities, *Commission Directive 2006/86/EC implementing Directive 2004/23/EC of the European Parliament and of the Council as regards traceability requirements, notification of serious adverse reactions and events and certain technical requirements for the coding, processing, preservation, storage and distribution of human tissues and cells (Text with EEA relevance)*, 2006, Oct 24.
89. Council, *Council Decision (1999/468/EC) laying down the procedures for the exercise of implementing powers conferred on the Commission*, 1999, Jun 28.
90. Council, *Council Decision (2006/512/EC) amending Decision 1999/468/EC laying down the procedures for the exercise of implementing powers conferred on the Commission*, 2006, Jul 17.
91. Article 29 Data Protection Working Party, WP155rev.04, *Working Document on Frequently Asked Questions (FAQs) related to Binding Corporate Rules, adopted on 24 June 2008, as last revised and adopted on 8 April 2009*, 2009, Apr 8.
92. Article 29 Data Protection Working Party, WP154, *Working Document Setting up a framework for the structure of Binding Corporate Rules*, 2008, Jun 24.
93. Article 29 Data Protection Working Party, WP153, *Working Document setting up a table with the elements and principles to be found in Binding Corporate Rules*, 2008, Jun 24.
94. Article 29 Data Protection Working Party, WP133, *Recommendation 1/2007 on the Standard Application for Approval of Binding Corporate Rules for the Transfer of Personal Data*, 2007, Jan 10.
95. Article 29 Data Protection Working Party, WP108, *Working Document Establishing a Model Checklist Application for Approval of Binding Corporate Rules*, 2005, Apr 14.
96. Article 29 Data Protection Working Party, WP107, *Working Document Setting Forth a Co-Operation Procedure for Issuing Common Opinions on Adequate Safeguards Resulting From "Binding Corporate Rules"*, 2005, Apr 14.
97. Article 29 Data Protection Working Party, WP74, *Working Document: Transfers of personal data to third countries: Applying Article 26 (2) of the EU Data Protection Directive to Binding Corporate Rules for International Data Transfers*, 2003, Jun 3.
98. Commission of the European Communities, *Commission Decision (2002/16/EC) on standard contractual clauses for the transfer of personal data to processors established in third countries, under Directive 95/46/EC (Text with EEA relevance)*, 2001, Dec 27.
99. Data Protection Unit of the Directorate – General for Justice, Freedom and Security at the European Commission, *Answers to Frequently Asked Questions Relating to Transfers of Personal Data From the EU/EEA to Third Countries*, 2009, Mar 17.
100. European Commission (Research Directorate-General, Directorate L – Science, Economy and Society, Unit L3 – Governance and Ethics), *Ethical Review in FP7 Guidance for Applicants, Informed Consent, http://cordis.europa.eu/fp7/home_en.html*, 2009, Dec 3.
101. Article 29 Data Protection Working Party, WP12, *Working Document: Transfers of personal data to third countries: Applying Articles 25 and 26 of the EU data protection directive*, 1998, Jul 24.

102. Commission of the European Communities, *Commission Decision (2001/497/EC), on standard contractual clauses for the transfer of personal data to third countries, under Directive 95/46/EC (Text with EEA relevance)*, 2001, Jun 15.
103. Commission of the European Communities, *Commission Decision (2004/915/EC), amending Decision 2001/497/EC as regards the introduction of an alternative set of standard contractual clauses for the transfer of personal data to third countries (Text with EEA relevance)*, 2004, Dec 27.
104. Commission of the European Communities, *Commission Staff Working Document, on the Implementation of the Commission decisions on standard contractual clauses for the transfer of personal data to third countries (2001/497/EC and 2002/16/EC)*, 2006, Jan 20.
105. Article 29 Data Protection Working Party, *WP34, Opinion 6/2000 on the Genome Issue*, 2000, Jul 13.

Index

Access Principles 38, 142
aCDB 189
AES 35, 54
AGN 40, 73, 189
anonymization 2, 4–7, 23, 24, 27, 29–35, 37, 39, 40–42, 67, 69, 70, 71, 73, 119, 120, 122, 123, 133, 134, 136, 137, 140–144, 146, 149, 150, 161
anonymized data 23, 3–41, 71, 123, 150, 163

barcode 31, 40, 72, 73, 120, 134–138, 140
BCR 189
BDSG 6, 7, 73, 143, 189
Binding Corporate Rules 76, 84–86, 99, 100–102
Biobanks Act 7
bSID 134, 138, 139, 189

CDI 30, 31, 33, 34, 40, 41, 122, 135, 136, 140, 189
CFR 43, 102, 104–106, 109, 112, 113, 146, 149, 164, 189
Change Control Management 57
Checklist 101, 129, 144–150
CIOMS 114, 131, 179, 189
clients 53
Clinical Trial Protocol 6, 40, 141, 148
clinical trials 1, 6, 26, 43, 48, 49, 76, 89, 111, 141, 144, 161, 163
COE 82, 127, 153, 157, 161, 169, 170–173, 189
Council of Europe 77, 78, 80, 127, 153, 157, 186
CRF 135, 136, 138, 140, 189
CRO 72, 73, 133–140, 145–148, 150, 189

Data Economy 39
data protection 1, 2, 21, 29, 33, 34, 37, 43, 67, 73, 74, 76, 78–80, 82–87, 90, 91, 93, 94, 97, 98, 100–102, 125, 140–148, 150, 153, 159, 162, 172, 185, 187, 188, 189
Data Reduction 39
Data Security 2, 120
Decisions 76, 77
Declaration of Helsinki 109, 131, 167
Decommissioning 58
Directives 76, 77
DNA 5, 7, 20, 40, 69, 72, 73, 76, 81, 114, 120, 133–137, 139, 143, 145–147, 159, 163, 177
dynamic variables 28

ECHR 77, 80, 153, 190
EC Treaty 88, 90
EEA 89, 90, 93–101, 145, 190
EMA 15, 76, 121, 127, 128, 161, 190
ePrivacy Directive 87, 90, 91, 155
Ethical Committee Restrictions 31, 32
Ethics Committees 2, 6, 31, 32, 40, 67, 115, 118, 121, 123, 124, 148, 149
EU Privacy Directive 21, 76, 82–90, 92–94, 97, 109, 110, 153, 157, 168, 185, 188
External Biobanking 140
external service 72, 73, 133, 143

FDA 43–45, 76, 102, 112, 121, 130, 190
Functional Requirements 48

GCP 1, 128, 190
GDI 30, 31, 34, 133–139, 189
GenDG 116, 181
genetic analysis 2, 3, 4, 26, 31, 32, 67, 69, 71, 117, 121, 124, 146, 159, 160, 170–173, 181, 182
genetic data 1, 2, 5–7, 20, 21, 28–30, 32, 34–36, 38, 39, 42, 67, 68, 70–72, 76, 89, 107, 113, 115, 116, 120, 122, 123, 140, 141, 145, 146, 150, 157–161, 172, 173, 178, 179, 187, 189
genetic IC 40, 116, 123, 148
genetic material 114, 122–124, 145, 177
genetic pattern 3, 4, 28
Genetic Review Board 6, 67, 71, 144, 150
genetic samples 23, 32, 114, 133, 181, 183
genotype 28
German Federal Data Protection Act 21
German National Ethics Council 7
GINA 107, 108, 190
Global Initiatives 130
Good Clinical Practice 1, 43, 111, 113
GRB 67–69, 71, 144, 189

hardware – servers 53
HIPAA 26, 105, 106, 107, 128, 129, 164, 190

ICH Guideline 43
identification 5, 28, 54, 123, 135–137, 139, 153, 157, 158, 161, 164, 165, 169

informed consent 2, 7, 26, 31, 33, 104, 109, 110, 111–118, 127, 129, 130, 144, 148, 149, 151, 166, 167, 174, 175, 176, 178, 179
Installation Qualification 44, 58
Institutional Review Board 31, 104, 107
International Declaration on Human Genetic Data 1, 116
IRB 32, 103, 107, 111, 129, 190

Key Protection Database 31, 34, 68, 69, 70, 73
key relationship 30, 31, 34, 40, 41, 70, 71
KPDB 31, 34, 40, 70–73, 133–136, 140, 189

Legal Requirements 2, 7
LIMS 39, 41, 145

masking 23–27, 29, 30
masking procedure 28, 29
masking rules 29, 33, 144, 149
MedDRA 35
medical data 20, 80, 81, 107, 115, 157, 158, 169–174, 186, 187
medical research 109, 121, 161, 174
monitoring 54

nCDI 34, 40, 41, 70, 71, 122, 189
nGDI 31, 34, 40, 41, 69, 70–73, 134, 135–137, 139, 147, 189

OECD 44, 46, 79, 80, 190
Operational Qualification 44, 51, 59, 61
Opinions 76, 77, 101, 127
Organizational Principle 39
Oviedo Convention 110, 174

P3G 7
Performance Qualification 44, 48, 60, 61
Periodic Review 58
PGx 41
pharmacogenetic results 15, 161
Prespecified Mode 3, 4, 5, 6, 117, 145
Pre- Unspecified Mode 3
Privacy Act 102, 107, 187
Problem Management 55
protection mask 17, 24, 38, 151, 161

QA 50

randomization 26, 179
rCDI 70, 71, 189
Recommendations 76, 77, 127, 162
Regulations 7, 76, 77, 102, 112, 113, 128, 129, 130, 162
Request Management 6, 34, 39, 67, 144, 150
Request Specification 68
Research Act 103
rGDI 70, 71, 72, 189
Risk Analysis 62, 64

Safe Harbor 96, 97, 129, 188
Screening Mode 3, 4, 117, 145
SDK 34, 67
SDLC 47, 58, 190
SDV 5, 6, 40, 148, 189
Security Management 53
Security Measures 37, 122
SGN 73, 189
SNOMED 35
SOPs 39, 62, 128
static variables 28
Storage Principles 38
Study Modes 3, 5, 24
Subrequest 71, 72
System Design Specification 50
System Programming 50

three entities approach 34, 67
Traceability 63, 64

UNESCO 116, 175, 190
UN - ICCPR 188
Unspecified Mode 4, 5, 6, 117, 145
User Requirements 48

validation 43–47, 51, 58, 60, 61, 65

WHO 35, 115, 179, 190
WHO-DD 35
withdrawal 33, 112, 115, 116, 122, 123, 149, 169, 175, 178
Working Party 83–86, 95, 96, 98, 100–102, 127, 129, 154, 155